# ULTRASOUND AND CANCER

# ULTRASOUND AND CANCER

Proceedings of the First International Symposium on Ultrasound and Cancer, Brussels, July 23–24, 1982 Invited papers and selected free communications

*Editor:*

**Salvator Levi**
*Ob. Gyn. Dept. (R. Vokaer)*
*Diagnostic Ultrasound Unit and F.R.E.S.E.R.H.*
*University Hospital Brugmann,*
*Brussels*

 1982

**Excerpta Medica, Amsterdam-Oxford-Princeton**

International Congress Series No. 587
ISBN Excerpta Medica 90 219 0587 6
ISBN Elsevier Science Publ. Co. 0 444 90270 8


**Library of Congress Cataloging in Publication Data**

International Symposium on Ultrasound and Cancer (1st :
    1982 : Brussels, Belgium)
    Ultrasound and cancer.
    Includes index.
    1. Cancer—Diagnosis—Congresses.  2. Diagnosis-
Ultrasonic—Congresses.  I. Levi, Salvator.  II. Title.
[DNLM: 1. Neoplasms—Diagnosis—Congresses.  2. Ultra-
sonics—Diagnostic use—Congresses.  W3 EX89 no. 587
1982  /  QZ 241 I605 1982u]
RC270.I495  1982  616.99'407543  82-9385
ISBN 0-444-90270-8 (Elsevier Science Pub. Co.)


*Publisher:*
**Excerpta Medica**
305 Keizersgracht
P.O. Box 1126
1000 BC Amsterdam

*Sole Distributors for the USA and Canada:*
**Elsevier Science Publishing Co., Inc.**
52 Vanderbilt Avenue
New York, NY 10017

Printed in The Netherlands by Casparie Amsterdam

# List of main authors

*Invited papers*

M. Afschrift, Belgium
J. Croll, Australia
L. Denis, Belgium
N. Frédéric, Belgium
B. Goldberg, U.S.A.
J. Jellins, Australia
G. Kossoff, Australia
A. Kratochwil, Austria
A. Kurjak, Yugoslavia
S. Levi, Belgium

K. Ossoinig, U.S.A.
M. Plainfosse, France
K. Sekiba, Japan
N. Spehl, Belgium
J. Thijssen, The Netherlands
T. Wagai, Japan
H. Watanabe, Japan
F. Weill, France
D. White, Canada


*Free papers*

Y. Bandai, Japan
M. Bazzocchi, Italy
J. Bruneton, France
L. Carlier, Belgium
W. Curati, Switzerland
F. Destro, Italy

A. Eisenscher, France
G. Maresca, Italy
R. Matallana, U.S.A.
W. Möckel, F.R.G.
G. Rizzatto, Italy
Y. Yasuda, Japan

---

We would like to express our sincere gratitude to Professor Henri Tagnon, Professor of Cancerology at the Université Libre de Bruxelles and President of the E.O.R.T.C., for accepting the Presidency of this Symposium.

Organizing Committee

# Preface

The diagnostic use of ultrasound energy and its properties has been increasingly developed over the past twenty-five years for an impressive variety of indications and for almost all medical specialties. With ultrasound techniques, the contours of superficial and deep structures in the body can be defined noninvasively and without harmful effects. Furthermore, their content and architecture can be characterized qualitatively. Active work is also in progress with a view to obtaining quantitative information. The feasibility to diagnose cancer, or at least to aid in diagnosing, has often been demonstrated but in a dispersed manner. The goal of the Symposium and of its published proceedings is to present collectively the actual results obtained in the endeavour to diagnose cancer with ultrasound. The survey of the methods and results is supplemented by discussion around the problems encountered when criteria corresponding to cancer lesions have to be defined. The problems arising from ultrasonic cancer detection and the diagnosis methods are seldom restricted to a limited field or specialty: most of the criteria used for cancer detection or tissue characterization are based on physical features related to sound-tissue interaction; they can be applicable, with some small differences, to the majority of human tissues. For those having diagnostic ultrasound as a primary interest, all subjects, all organs or fields are of interest. For the others, more involved in only one specialty, knowledge about the use of some methods developed for diagnosing cancer in other, more or less restricted areas, is worthwhile and could give invaluable information if applicable on their own. The reasons to gather, under the common denomination Ultrasound and Cancer, chapters related to many different organs and functions are thus more obvious.

This book contains invited papers reporting the experience of diagnostic ultrasound practitioners; most of them have a worldwide reputation due to their outstanding merit and valuable contribution to the progress in diagnosic ultrasound, and due to their first-class publications and presentations. Diagnostic ultrasound started quite early in Belgium — in 1966 the Editor was among the few using A-mode and then B-mode ultrasound in Europe — and to hold such a Symposium in Brussels was an opportunity to become acquainted with some skilled Belgian ultrasonologists who have good experience in cancer diagnosis.

A call for papers from various authors concerned with Ultrasound and Cancer was made with a view to ensuring a wide and comprehensive coverage of the subject and, after an inevitable selection, to avoiding duplication as far as possible. The readers of this book will have the invaluable advantage of the very short interval between the preparation of the manuscripts and the publication of the proceedings: they are published at the time of the public presentation of the papers. Support and criticisms are welcome for improving the next, II International Symposium on Ultrasound and Cancer.

The Editor

# Foreword

Does ultrasonography help, facilitate or allow to give a precise diagnosis in the field of oncology, whatever may be the organ or tissue involved in the cancerous process?

This will be asked to the participants of the 'First International Symposium on Ultrasound and Cancer' held in Brussels the 23rd and 24th July 1982, organized by Salvator Levi, M.D., head of the Unité de Diagnostic par Ultrasons de la Clinique Obstétricale et Gynécologique de l'Hôpital Universitaire Brugmann and supported by the European Organization for Research on Treatment of Cancer and the Belgian Society of Diagnostic Ultrasound.

The subject is ambitious and one can ask why such a symposium covering all aspects of oncologic ultrasonography is promoted by gynecologists. The reason is, that in our department, S. Levi started to study, ten years ago, how to characterize tissue texture in vivo, noninvasively, in order to elucidate − or trying to do so − the nature of pelvic or abdominal masses. At that time, with the help of a commercially available equipment, S. Levi gathered interesting results presented for the first time in 1974 at the Institut de Génie Biologique et Médicale de Vandoeuvre (France): 'Essai d'Analyse Quantitative des Echogrammes de Tumeurs Pelviennes'. The results were encouraging enough to carry on the experiments with more sophisticated method, granted by the Fonds National de la Recherche Scientifique and the Fonds Lequime-Ropsy.

Later, J. Keuwez, Physicist, joined Dr S. Levi's team. The computerization of acquired ultrasonic signals combined to the automation of scanning are now in progress.

The Fondation pour la Recherche en Endocrinologie Sexuelle et l'Etude de la Reproduction Humaine (F.R.E.S.E.R.H.) supported Dr Levi's work in order to carry on his original experiments, with the aid of the new tools, because of the interest brought to the work, more particularly in the U.S.A. where he received the title of Senior Research Scientist from the Indianapolis Center for Advanced Research. The Department of Physical and Natural Sciences of the Commission of the European Communities also became interested and concluded in 1977 a research contract with our ultrasound laboratory.

The noninvasive, in vivo, analysis of tissue texture, appears to be promising for all kind of tumors in the whole body: therefore the F.R.E.S.E.R.H. and the OB-GYN Department of the Université Libre de Bruxelles, support as much as possible the research of ultrasound in cancer diagnosis.

Prof. R. Vokaer
Chef de la Clinique Obstétricale et Gynécologique
de l'Hôpital Universitaire Brugmann (U.L.B.).
Administrateur-Directeur de la F.R.E.S.E.R.H.

# Introduction

Our subject today is ultrasound and cancer. More specifically what is the contribution of the ultrasound technic to the diagnosis and treatment of human cancer. The answer to this important question will be given by the speakers of this symposium brilliantly organized by Dr Salvator Levi and sponsored by the service of gynecology and obstetrics of the University of Brussels.

We oncologists are often asked 'when will the cancer problem be solved?' The answer to this question is that it is being solved every day, progressively like all medical problems. The year 1981 marked the tenth anniversary of the *National Cancer Act* of the Government of the U.S.A. which dramatically put the emphasis on a renewed and expanded effort to study and advance the treatment of cancer in the U.S.A. This is the country which has a real vision of science. We all here have confidence in the scientific method, whether applied to clinical studies and in the laboratory. Good work and discoveries come from every country from all parts of the world but especially from countries which make good use of their intellectual potential. The man who signs a paper describing an important discovery is indebted to all humanity past and present for over 99% of the ingredients of the discovery. We in Belgium should be thankful to countries with vision.

What are some of the important advances of the last 10 years in terms of practical results, leaving out for today's occasion the tremendous explosion of biological laboratory research which prepares an even brighter future: in children, long-term survival increased from less than 10% to over 50%. By 1980 many of our children patients have become healthy adults and have families of their own. It would be instructive to analyze in detail the many factors which have contributed to this victory, among which should be noted first the development of cytotoxic chemotherapy to the point that chemotherapy became a full partner, with radiotherapy and surgery, for the care of cancer. We all realize of course that the problem of curing cancer is bound to this strange property of cancer to metastasize and more often than not to metastasize before the primary is or can be detected.

Therefore, treatment addressed to local disease to the exclusion of systemic treatment rarely achieves cure and then only in specific cases. This is well exemplified by breast cancer in which any type of operation with or without radiotherapy produces the equivalent rate of *failures*, amounting to over 70 to 80%. Therefore a systemic treatment appears indispensable and physicians who scorn at chemotherapeutic research should remember this and assist in finding other modilities of systemic treatment, perhaps chemotherapeutic, perhaps of different types, some of which are of immense interest and cannot be discussed here.

Not only in children but also in adults has systemic treatment in the form of chemotherapy following local treatment by X-ray given gratifying results: Hodgkin's disease (70% survival at 10 years), lymphosarcoma, testicular tumors (over 90% cures with certain regimen), many others. These tumors had a very high mortality as recently as 20 years ago.

There is a second factor: the development of improved radiotherapy and especially of chemotherapy would have been impossible without the parallel development of a precise and reliable methodology for the evaluation of clinical results. Such development is necessary in all fields of clinical medicine but nowhere more than in cancer medicine. Cancer therapy, cancer cure is the repository of the hopes of mankind and represents the supreme temptation for the honest physician to mistake his hopes for reality. Hence the vagaries and the unreliability of early clinical investigation in cancer therapy. The important present day evolution is the advent and generalization of the controlled clinical trial.

One of the sponsors of this meeting is the European Organization for Research on Treatment of Cancer. It is a non-governmental organization which comprises the most important cancer hospitals and research centers in Western Europe. It is not a society in the usual sense, but it is a working association to promote clinical groups for the clinical evaluation of the new treatments created in the laboratories. There are over 1500 participating physicians in 150 hospitals and clinics. 9000 patients per year are registered and treated according to carefully worked out and detailed protocols of treatment uniformly applied. The results are assembled in a 'Data Center' located in Brussels. There the data managers supervise the normal flow of incoming results from the participating hospitals; the statisticians verify the validity of the conclusions. Quality of life and ethical obligations are also studied and strictly supervised. The clinical trials of the E.O.R.T.C., working hand in hand with similar organizations in the U.S.A., are an irreplaceable instrument for progress in cancer treatment.

I now realize that I should say something about ultrasound and cancer. I will tell you that we in the Cancer Center of Institut Jules Bordet and our radiological department like the ultrasound technic and apply it extensively. Dr Levi who is a pioneer in this field and the founder of the Society deserves our admiration and gratitude. However the speakers in this symposium are the ones who know much on ultrasound and I now shall let them tell you their story.

Prof. H.J. Tagnon
President, E.O.R.T.C.

# Contents

## 4. Pelvis

## 5. Retroperitoneum

# IMPEDIMENTS IN TISSUE CHARACTERIZATION FOR CANCER DIAGNOSIS

Salvator Levi and José Keuwez

*Ultrasound Laboratory, Department of Gynecology and Obstetrics, University Hospital Brugmann, 1020 Brussels, Belgium*

## I. INTRODUCTION

Ultrasonography is an imaging technique based on the reflection, by the human body, of sound pulses. Sound penetrates into the body, interacts with the encountered tissues. Sound tissue interactions have name scattering, absorption, refraction and diffusion. Reflected sounds are received back by the emitting transducer during its long non-emitting periods. Special technical procedures display into an image the received signals arising from the insonified area. Spatial display and relative intensity of echoes constitute the basement of echography and diagnosis.

A diagnosis is suggested through the interpretation of image, based on sound-tissue interaction. Only a few facets of interaction are taken into account: mainly the backscattering and the attenuation because they may strongly alter the echo-formed image. However, the basic information is mainly morphological, qualitative, somewhat quantitative but rather subjective.

As mentionned above, the sound wave is disturbed by various mechanisms. If their respective contribution to disturbances is different from tissue to tissue and from a healthy tissue to its pathological state, the quantification of these mechanisms and of their combinations, should constitute the acoustical signature of a given tissue.

When a catalog of signatures from the different human tissues will be available, as well in normal as in different pathological conditions,diagnoses of diseases affecting the properties of tissues will be made through the determination and identification of their signatures.

Everybody forecasts that the main hope put into ultrasound tissue characterization is related to the possible ability to perform non-invasive "biopsies". Sonic biopsy is a sampling of ultrasonic information which has to be analyzed in order to distinguish objectively and accurately between benign and malignant lesions.

1

## II. BASIC CONCEPTS

### PHYSICS

**Sound waves** are mechanical waves, energy which propagates into a medium, human tissues for example. That energy is partly **reflected** to the transducer: this is the fundamental phenomenon which produces signals and then an image or **echogram.**

**Reflection** occurs where sound waves pass trough the **interface** of two media. Reflection is strong, more especially as the media impedances are different (impedance = product of **density** and **sound velocity**).

The **transmitted energy** (i.e.the non-reflected part), somewhat **refracted,** is damaged by a serie of sound-tissue interactions: a.**scattering,** or spreading of the energy by non-uniformities in the medium, even particles smaller than one wavelenght; b.**friction forces:** a part of the wave energy is transformed into heat. The resultant of wave damages is called **attenuation,** which appears to be easier to measure than any of its components. Therefore, determination of attenuation could be one of the best approach for tissue characterization by ultrasound (UTC).

### CHARACTERIZATION BASED ON IMAGE

To a certain extent, UTC is feasible on images. **History of ultrasound imaging** for the past 12 years could be summarized into three stages:

1. Interest for A-Mode trace as well as the possibility to display it have diminished. This is explained by the fact that A-Mode traces are rather difficult to interpret, despite the fact they contain much information.

2. Grey-tones images have supplanted the black and white where all printed dots are equally bright, whatever their amplitude is. The only condition to appear on the echogram is to reach a predetermined level of amplitude. Grey-tones (8 to 64) display more information. Grey-tone image permits a visual characterization, very subjective, non-quantitative. Its quality depends, between many other factors, on sound **frequency** which acts on **resolution,** on scanning mode (simple scan, compound, with or without **overwriting**), on the different settings and on equipment.

3. Beside static B-Scan, dynamic B-Scan or real-time imaging, contributes specifically to make better diagnosis. Real time has two main advantages: easy handling and detection of movements. For example, a bowel loop cannot be interpreted as an ovarian or salpinx cyst lesion if peristaltic movements are detected. Abnormal movements could also be a powerful aid for diagnosis. The immobility of an organ compared to the others can be a sign of adherences. They are also important features which restricts sometimes its use (1).

# IMAGE FEATURES OF TISSUES

Many influences - some of them out of control - modify the aspect of images, but careful observation bring valuable information on the particular nature of some tissues. **Adipose tissue** is an organized compound fat and fibrous tissue producing non-, low- and strong echoic areas. The image texture is characteristic of that adipose tissue (Fig.1). Between fat and muscle, **aponevrosis** reflects very well ultrasounds. **Muscles** are irregularly echogenic. **Bones** reflect sounds highly, thus transmitted energy is very low; they are almost perfect reflectors. On the borderline of gas containing tissues - **lungs, bowels** - sounds are reflected and penetrate a few; gas bubbles scatter the transmitted energy. Homogeneous liquids do not reflect neither scatter sounds (Fig.1,2,3). Secretions, exsudates and transsudates, filtration products, urine, gall, ascitis, are homogeneous liquids in normal conditions. As sound velocity is lower in liquids than in tissues, sound-attenuation is also weaker and refractions could be more important (2). Low attenuation and refraction have some effects on image: echo-amplitude enhancement at distal part of liquid area and shadowing on its lateral edges.

Blood is not visualized but scatters ultrasound: indeed circulating blood is detected by Doppler effect. Blood is acoustically comparable to other tissues: density and sound velocity are equivalent to those of the liver: 1.06 and 1560 m/sec respectively. **Other liquids** as pus, sebaceous substance in teratomas, may have a marked scattering effect and are more attenuating than water. **Liver, pancreas, spleen, placenta** and **fetal lung tissue** contain many very small size reflectors which are responsible for typical echograms, with regularly distributed echoes of even amplitude. Echo-distribution is only disturbed by "foreign" structures belonging to the organ: vessels and excretory canals for example. Some physiological factors can modify echodistribution and echoamplitude (placenta ageing, fetal lung maturity) as well as pathological ones (inflammation, calcification, fibrosis, infarcts, ...).
The contrasts between the organs or between tissues in the organ may be enhanced by fat tissue and liquids (Fig.3). Foreign bodies and wall abnormalities (of stomach, gallbladder, urinary bladder) may be seen, even if their size is very small (ulcus, papillary tissue, small tumors). Visualization of these is greatly improved by the contrast brought by liquids (acoustical window) and therefore better studied by characterization techniques. Oedema and blood infiltration into tissues modify also their image. Calcium deposits may produce high reflections but the size of calcification is predominent for absorption as for reflection and/or scattering.

The peculiarities of the image, when they are correctly described and interpreted - with a good knowledge of the technical conditions applied for echogram building - are

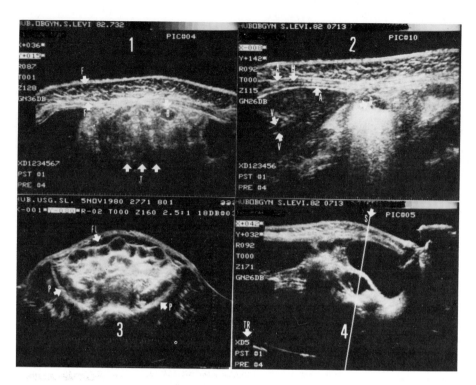

*Figure* 1. Longitudinal scan of the abdomen. Skin and adipose tissue lie between the two arrows F. Under muscles and aponevrosis, bowels loop are visible (B); sound energy is not transmitted to the spine because attenuation by gazes (arrows T).

*Figure* 2. Abdominal wall layers, liver and duodenum (D); A = aponevrosis, M = muscles, V = vessel within the liver.

*Figure* 3. Ascitis and bowels filled with liquid (transverse scan); FL = fluid, P = pelvic bones.

*Figure* 4. Pelvic tumor submitted to sonic biopsy. The line of sight (S),from which samples are collected, is the axis of the transducer 5 (TR) (All the pictures were tooken on U.I.Octoson).

informatory enough to give or approach a precise diagnosis. Sonar information have to be added to other collected data (anamnesis,physical examination ...), to knowledge of anatomy, physiology and pathology, all factors which are to be harmoniously integrated in the brain mechanisms leading to diagnosis. Diagnosis approach,as described above, gives very satisfactory results on a statistical point of vue, very close to the real situation in most of cases.

Analysis of transmitted energies could be added to analysis of reflection. Very useful **in vitro** in order to determine most of the acoustical parameters of tissues, it appears presently to be much less applicable **in vivo**. Indeed, transmission does not bring any information on the localization of studied interactions and is very often too weak because sound penetration is difficult throughout the whole human body (Fig.1,2).

Yet, image is sometimes not informative enough to chose between different situations and to decide for one conclusion with an acceptable risk of error. The space occupied by the uncertain diagnoses, when image may fit with many different lesions, could certainly be reduced if the evaluation of sound tissue interactions could be approach differently and by priority by quantitative ultrasonic tissue characterization to differentiate between normal, benign and malignant tissues.

## III.OBJECTIVE AND QUANTITATIVE MEANS TO CHARACTERIZE TISSUES

A.**Pattern recognition**: The image represents only a limited part of the echographic information (mapping, signals levels). Moreover, the sonologist perceives it only in a restrictive and subjective way.
An automatic image-processing can present objectively to the sonologist a deal of the imperceivable information: as for example, the echo-density and its distribution. Analysis could be performed on the raw image; it can also be performed on an image modified either to accentuate some of its features,or to extract information which could hide other. These techniques were applied successfully to improve the diagnosis of prostatic cancerous diseases (3).
B. The **Doppler effect** is effective to determine blood flow in vessels, even quantitatively using pulsed sounds. Texture changes may induce modifications of blood flow, especially in breast cancer. The tissue infiltrations is followed by increase of blood flow in the abnormal breast compared to the heterolateral breast. The Doppler effect could be useful in the detection and identification of breast tumors but also for other organs (4) : the tumoral part of a pancreas shows different Doppler signals than the normal part.
C.Cancer affects the **elasticity and compressibility** properties of tissues; the response to external forces is modified. Moreover when cancerous and peripheral tissues

are submitted to mechanical oscillation, the cancerous tissues respond differently. This method, named echosysmography (5), has been tested on liver, pancreatic, renal tumors and accessorily could be useful for breast investigations.

### D.Sound-tissues interactions

a)Velocity: sound velocity measured by transmission techniques is different in normal and cancerous parts of various organs, as it has been shown **in vitro** for hepatic and breast tissues. This change has a special interest for **in vivo** examination of breast, better adapted to transmission method than other structures. Maps of velocities profiles in the breast can be constructed (6).

b)Scattering: the backscattered energy is dependent on the frequency and structure of the medium. The structure may be modified by some diseases. Trials were made to detect changes in the backscattered energy to diagnose liver and thyroid anomalies (7). This approach would be interesting for early detection of pathology because scattering could be modified before attenuation.

c)Attenuation: much attention has been focused on the attenuation of sound energy to characterize tissues. Attenuation was evaluated on echograms and the first practical applications were made by the Japanase School. The **graded tomography** (8,9) is a quantitative evaluation of attenuation. Although approximative, it gives a surprising high rate of correct diagnosis in breast cancer. The increase of attenuation with frequency is a property of sounds used for **in vivo** characterization (10). Noteworthly results were obtained for the differentiation of liver diseases (11) by **spectral analysis.** A similar method is under development in our laboratory.

The central part of the amplitude spectrum, of a pulsed sound wave, has the shape of a gaussian curve. The modification of this part with depth penetration is the mark of the various interactions, already described during the propagation in the medium. The characteristics of the decrease of the amplitudes are supposed to characterize the medium.

The amplitude spectrum of echoes, arising from two reflectors located on the same pathway, are compared with the aim to calculate the attenuation in the medium. One single value obtained by this comparison is not representative of the attenuation by the medium. Attenuation can be determined only from the distribution of these values. Significant differences between spectra are obtained when the distance between echoes of each pair is large enough. But when the distance becomes to long, the points generating the echoes are not similarly perceived by the transducer. Indeed, the shape of the sound field changes with the depth. The best appropriate distance depends on frequency and attenuation of the medium. The use of high frequencies allows to reduce the distance and to characterize smaller structures. However, with high frequencies, the attenuation in the intervening tissues is burdensome for the measurements.

To insure the independance of the samples, sampling should

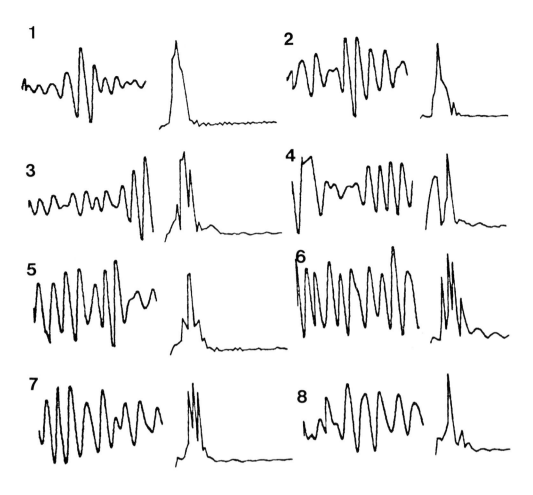

*Figure* 5. A window is displaced along the transducer output and
signals from tissues digitized by a transient digitizer and stored
on storage media. The corresponding amplitude spectra shows important variation in amplitude due to various effects such phase
cancellations. The usefull information to characterize tissues
should be extracted by a statistical method.

fulfill some requirements. Parallel propagation axes and non-overlapping fields ensure the independance of the samples. Under these conditions, the method may be adequate to determine a coefficient for attenuation. Nevertheless, the estimated coefficient and the true value of attenuation may be different, but the goal will be reached when the differentiation of tissues will be realized.

In the practice, the area to be analyzed is first localized on the image produced by an automatic ultrasonic scanner (U.I.Octoson). This machine is particularly well adapted to conduct such experimentations. Eight transducers are fastened on a nacel mobile along the three orthogonal axes (i.e.in any direction). Furthermore, each transducer effects a sector scan (adjustable angles). The displacement of transducers are monitored through a console and parallel propagation paths are easily obtained. The output of any selected transducer is fed to a computer (Digital PDP 11/44) through a transient digitizer and then transferred to storage media for post-processing (Fig.4,5).

## IV.CONCLUSIONS

As far as we know, **no decisive** method exists which allows to distinguish between normal tissues neither to differentiate their normal and pathological states. The problem is still to be solved and effective method to perform the ultrasonic tissue characterization are not obvious at all. However, there is no doubt about the imagination and the ressources put in this endeaviour. Nevertheless, the goal should be reached and should step over the differentiation of begnin and malignant tissues or between various pathological stages only by observation of the image.

Fundamental and clinical research on tissue characterization must be promoted, as a potientially important and supplementary non-invasive tool to fight against cancer. Diagnostic ultrasound evolves to complete its morphological information by functionnal (blood flow, movements, filling, voiding,...) diagnosis and by analysis tissue structure and content. It should even be foreseen that the different ways to diagnose with ultrasound could be followed during a single examination session. This is the (next ?) future.

## REFERENCES

1. **S.LEVI, J.KEUWEZ:** "New trends in diagnostic ultrasound: medico-technological aspects" In: Real-Time Ultrasound in Perinatal Medicine (ed.R.Chef), S.Karger, Basel, volume 6, p.129-138, 1979.
2. **P.N.T.WELLS:** "Basic Physics" In: Handbook of Clinical Ultrasound, (eds.M.de Vlieger, J.Holmes, E.Kazner, G.Kossoff, A.Kratochwil, R.Kraus, J.Poujol and D.Strandness), John Wiley & Sons, New York, p.15-23, 1978.
3. **G.WESSELS, W.SEELEN, U.SCHEIDING:** "The application of pattern recognition in ultrasonic sectional pictures of

the prostate (B-Mode analysis)" In: Ultrasonic Tissue Characterization (ed.J.M.Thijssen), Stafleu's Scient.Publ.Comp., p.273-280, 1980.

4. **P.N.T..WELLS, M.HALLIWELL, R.MOUNTFORD:** "Tumour detection by ultrasonic Doppler blood-flow signals" In: Ultrasonic Tissue Characterization II (ed.M.Linzer), NBS Special Publication 525, p.173-176, 1979.

5. **EISENSCHER A.:** "Echosismography: a new method for tissue characterization" Excerpta Medica, Amsterdam, ICS 547, n.33 p14, 1981.

6. **G.GLOVER:** "Characterization of in vivo breast tissue by ultrasonic, time-of-flight computed tomography" In: Ultrasonic Tissue Characterization II (ed.M.Linzer), NBS Special Publication 525, p.221-225, 1979.

7. **NICHOLAS D.:** "An introduction to the theory of acoustic scattering by biological tissues. In: Recent Advances in Ultrasound in Biomedicine, Chapter 1 (ed.D.N.White), Research Studies Press.

8. **WAGAI T., TSUTSUMI M., TAKEUCHI H.:** "Diagnostic ultrasound in breast diseases". In: Present and Future of Diagnostic Ultrasound (eds.I.Donald and S.Levi), Kooyker Scient.Public., Rotterdam, p.148-161, 1976.

9. **T.KOBAYASHI, O.TAKATANI, N.HATTORI, K.KIMURA:** "Differential diagnosis of breast tumors: sensitivity graded method of ultrasonotomography and clinical evaluation of its diagnostic accuracy", Cancer 33: 940-951, 1974.

10. **LEVI S., KEUWEZ J.:** "Tissue characterization in vivo by differential attenuation measurements" In: Ultrasonic Tissue CharacterizationII (ed.M.Linzer), NBS Special Publication 525, p.121-124, 1979.

11. **KUC R.:** "Clinical application of an ultrasound attenuation coefficient estimation technique for liver pathology characterization" IEEE Transactions on Biomedical Engineering 27: 312-319, 1980.

**Review**
**CHIVERS R.C.:** "Tissue Characterization" Ultrasound in Med. & Biol. Vol.7, p.1-20, 1981

# THE ROLE OF COMPUTERS IN ULTRASOUND CANCER DIAGNOSIS - VELOCITY MEASUREMENT TECHNIQUES

G. Kossoff

*Ultrasonics Institute, Sydney, NSW, Australia*

The development of grey scale echography and the resultant ability to study the internal texture of soft tissue organs allowed a major advance to be made in the detection and diagnosis of cancer. The spatial and contrast resolution of modern B-mode imaging equipment is now very good and is beginning to approach some of the theoretical limits. Indeed it is possible that in the next few years only refinements in performance will be attained and major advances in imaging may have to await the development of successful ultrasonic contrast agents.

Ultrasound today can detect malignancies with a specificity in the high 80% and a sensitivity in the mid 90%. This is an impressive achievement based on the qualitative assessment of only one acoustic parameter of tissue namely, the acoustic impedance discontinuity. A second acoustic parameter, attenuation, is portrayed indirectly by appearances such as shadowing or enhancement. Velocity is ignored and is considered a degrading factor as it smears the spatial resolution of compound scans. Of the information resident in the echo scattering cross-section only the direct back-scattered energy is employed and no attempt is made to display the acoustic impedance of tissue. Doppler has been used for some time for the study of blood flow. More recently it has been also used for imaging but as yet has not been used for cancer diagnosis. It would seem therefore that there is considerable scope for improvement through the development of tissue characterisation techniques which will allow the quantitative measurement of these acoustic parameters of tissue and their dependence on the nature of the interogating ultrasonic beam and the physiological activity of the tissues. Modern technical advances are strongly linked to the employment of sophisticated digital signal processing techniques, and computers will undoubtedly play a central role in improvements in ultrasonic diagnosis. The use of computers must however be cost effective. It is important therefore to identify the limitations of the simple B-mode imaging technique so as to set appropriate goals. Ideally the newly developed technique should also be able to be applied to a relatively large range of clinical conditions.

In cancer diagnosis account must also be taken that ultrasound is a tomographic procedure and the examination of a whole organ requires taking many sections. The method is therefore inherently not suitable for screening applications and is best applied to the examination of high risk patients.

Some of the limitations of the B-mode imaging technique which are potentially achievable goals by ultrasonic diagnosis lie in the following areas:

1. Distinguishing fat from other soft tissues. This is particularly important in the breast where fat and malignancies are portrayed as areas of low level echoes.
2. Differentiation between cystic and solid masses when the former such as abscesses contain internal echoes and the latter such as lymphomas are nearly echo-free.
3. Distinction between and identification of normal, benign and malignant tissues.
4. Detection of disseminated cancer affecting the whole organ. Because of the total involvement of the organ such malignancies are displayed by an uniform texture.
5. Identification of different types of biological liquids such as urine, free blood and ascites which on imaging are displayed as echo-free areas.

Although it is unreasonable to expect that all these limitations will be overcome in the near future, progress is gradually being achieved towards the attainment of these goals and this paper will discuss transmission and reflection techniques that have been developed so far for the quantitative measurement of velocity of propagation of ultrasound in tissues.

The velocity in fat is nearly 10% slower than in other soft tissues and a relatively coarse measurement of this parameter with techniques which can be applied in a clinical setting will allow the identification of fat from other tissues. The velocity in liquids is generally several percent less than that in soft tissues and a more accurate measurement technique should allow cystic/solid mass differentiation. The velocity in most soft tissues varies by a few percent and an accurate measurement technique should be able to characterise some of the normal, benign and malignant tissues. Changes due to increased fibrosis and fatty infiltration cause the velocity to increase or decrease respectively. Measurement of velocity could therefore diagnose the presence of such and other disseminated changes and allow the quantified determination of the degree of the infiltration. Finally, due to the varying protein and salt content, the velocity of ultrasound differs by one or two percent in the various biological liquids. Thus an accurate measuring technique could also identify various different liquids.

Ultrasound transmission reconstruction techniques similar to those employed in X-ray computerised tomography have been used for some time to provide quantitative images of velocity and attenuation in tissues. The computer is an essential component of the instrumentation and, as illustrated in Figure 1, these techniques are beginning to provide vital quantified information on the value of these acoustic parameters in living normal, benign and malignant tissues[1]. Reconstruction techniques are prone to an undershoot artifact following transition into a media with slow velocity. The low value for velocity in subcutaneous fat shown in the Figure is possibly affected by this artifact following transition from the relatively fast water coupling medium into the slower fat.

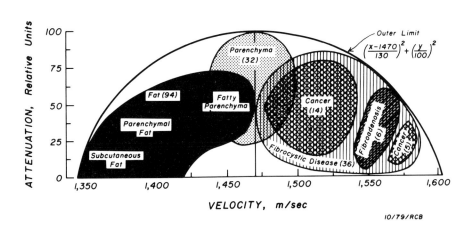

Figure 1. Velocity and attenuation of ultrasound in breast tissue. (Courtesy Dr J. Greenleaf, Mayo Foundation, Rochester, Minnesota)

Unfortunately, with the exception of the breast, few of the important organs in the body can be examined by transmission techniques. Also, due to the difficulties created by aberration in the propagating characteristics of the ultrasonic beam by the varying velocities of the constituent tissues, the quality of the ultrasonic transmission images does not match that obtained by the conventional B-mode technique. It is possible therefore that even in the breast the use of transmission imaging is likely to be complementary to the B-mode technique which would be used to determine areas of interest whilst the transmission image would then be used to quantify this area. For example difficulty is sometimes encountered in distinguishing between fatty infiltration and malignancy by the B-mode technique as both areas are portrayed as areas of low level echoes. The ability to determine the velocity in that area, low for fat, fast for malignancy, would be of considerable assistance in the differentiation.

An early example of the foreshadowed application is illustrated by Figure 2 which is a UI Octoson scan of a 37 year old patient with a palpable mass clinically considered to be a fibroadenoma. The echogram illustrates the presence of a 3cm mass. The lesion contains internal echoes, is encapsulated by a prominent anterior and posterior boundary, shows no attachments to the surrounding tissues and on simple scans was seen to cast a posterior shadow. All of these features are consistent with the B-mode appearance of a fibroadenoma but do not totally exclude the possibility of an uncommon malignancy or of a lipoma.

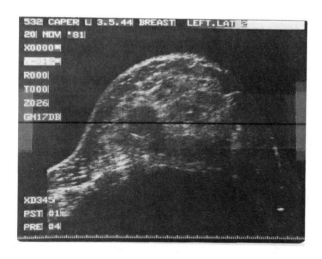

Figure 2. Echogram obtained on UI Octoson of a patient with a 3cm mass lesion. (Courtesy Royal Brisbane Hospital, University of Queensland)

14

A velocity reconstruction image obtained on equipment being developed by the Queensland Institute of Technology[2] at the level indicated on the echogram is shown in Figure 3. The black rim represents the subcutaneous fat in which, due to undershoot artifact, the velocity was calculated to be 1350m/sec. The average velocity in the breast parenchyma measures 1470m/sec suggesting considerable fatty infiltration. This is consistent with the B-mode image where the infiltration is portrayed by areas of low level echoes in the parenchyma. The lesion is clearly visualised as a white area at six o'clock. The velocity in the lesion was measured as 1530m/sec definitively excluding a lipoma from the differential diagnosis. On biopsy the lesion proved to be a fibroadenoma. Equipment combining reflection and transmission reconstruction imaging techniques in the same instrument is currently under development and the potential synergistic clinical usefulness of the two imaging techniques should become known in the not too distant future.

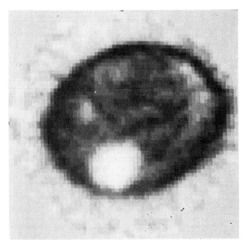

Figure 3. Velocity transmission reconstruction image in same patient. (Courtesy Queensland Institute of Technology.

Measurement of velocity based on reflection data is considerably more attractive as such a technique may be applied to all parts of the body capable of being examined by the B-mode technique. Recent studies undertaken at our Institute have demonstrated that the velocity measurements may be obtained by computer processing of data obtained from compound scans[3]. The studies were undertaken on the UI Octoson which with its structure of eight transducers in accurately defined spatial positions and a stand off water coupling path of known velocity forms an ideal instrument for such measurements. The principle of the technique is illustrated schematically in Figure 4. The examined object is scanned using one of the transducers and the simple scan echogram is stored in the computer. If the velocity in the object differs from that in the water coupling path, then due to refraction the ultrasonic beam is deviated in the object and echoes are obtained from impedance discontinuities along this deviated path. The equipment is however unaware of this deviation and plots the echoes as though they were being received along the line of sight of the transducer, i.e. in incorrect anatomical position. The object is then examined using another transducer and the second scan is also stored in the computer. Refraction again affects the positions in which structures are displayed and because different lines of sight are employed the structures are displayed in positions different to those obtained in the first scan, i.e. they fail to superimpose. The developed technique relies on identifying the same structure on the two echograms and measuring the degree of lack of superimposition. This information is then combined with the shape of the water/object interface obtained from the B-mode image to measure by cross-correlation techniques the velocity in the object.

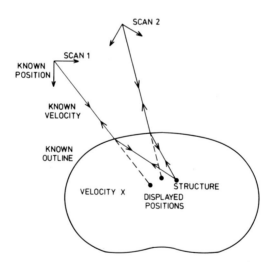

Figure 4 Principle of measurement of velocity by cross correlation of two simple scans. The scans are cross correlated to superimpose the position of the displayed echo from the same structure.

The method was tested using a phantom consisting of a cylindrical tank and a central wire containing a liquid of known velocity. The phantom was immersed in the UI Octoson and velocity determinations were made using the location of the central wire. Figure 5 is a double exposure of two simple scans of the phantom. The echoes from the central wire do not superimpose and the two lines of sight used for the measurement of the position of the central wire are illustrated. The contour of the phantom which was manually inputted into the computer with a trackball is also illustrated. Measurements were performed using different transducer pairs and averaging of the data allowed determination of velocity in the phantom to within 3 m/sec.

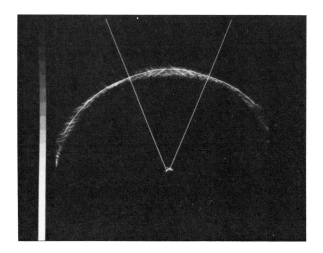

Figure 5. Echogram of cylinder with central wire phantom used for validation of cross correlation velocity measurement technique. Velocity in water/alcohol coupling medium 1555m/sec, in phantom 1600 m/sec.

The technique has also been applied to measure the velocity in larger organs such as the liver using the same two velocity model. In tissue no ideal point target is available and some internal feature such as a duct which is visible on a number of scans with different transducers is employed. Figure 6 is an example of two such simple scans. The contour of the abdominal wall was again manually inputted into the computer and measurements were performed averaging the results obtained using different transducer pairs. Comparison of results obtained at different depths and in different planes gave results which showed a variation of less than 15 m/sec. The velocity in the liver in normal patients measured by this method was found to be 1575 m/sec agreeing closely with the values obtained using conventional techniques recently published in the literature[4].

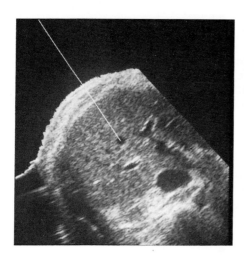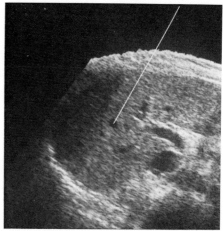

Figure 6. Two simple scans portraying same duct used in the cross correlation analysis. The shift in the two images corresponds to 1 and 3 pixels in horizontal and vertical co-ordinates respectively. The velocity in water/alcohol coupling medium is 1570 m/sec. The velocity in the liver measures 1575 m/sec.

Studies are in progress to develop techniques for use on a number of regions with different velocities. The velocity of the superficial layer may be determined using relatively shallow targets and successively deeper targets can then be examined using rays traversing regions with different velocities. Another approach is to utilise a number of regions deep in the tissue and carry out iterative reconstruction technique similar to tomographic reconstruction to solve for all velocities simultaneously. As a high quality cross-sectional image is already available from the B-mode data the precision and spatial resolution of the velocity determination need not be as great, simplifying the processing requirement. A system such as this could for example be adequate to provide the differential diagnosis between malignant regions and fatty inclusions in which there is a marked difference in velocity and where a coarse measurement is adequate.

In summary computers are starting to play a major role in extending the range of ultrasonic diagnosis. Apart from permitting more sophisticated processing of

18

the conventional ultrasonic data they are beginning to
allow the quantified measurement of other acoustic
parameters of tissue and thus the attainment of genuine
tissue characterisation. Because of its effectiveness
the B-mode imaging technique will remain the primary
ultrasonic examination procedure. Tissue
characterisation studies will be based on the
information provided by this technique such as the
determination of smaller areas of interest in the total
image and of the geometry of structures. Analysis of
the more limited areas with a coarser spatial resolution
requirement will allow less powerful computers to be
employed thus making tissue characterisation studies
more cost effective.

REFERENCES
1. Greenleaf, J.F. and Bahn, R.C. Clinical Imaging
   with Transmissive Ultrasonic Computerized
   Tomography. IEEE Transactions on Biomedical
   Engineering. BME-28, 177-185, February 1982.

2. Koch, R., Whiting, J.F., Price, D.C. and McCaffrey,
   J.F. Ultrasonic Computer Assisted Tomography of the
   Breast. Australasian Physical and Engineering
   Sciences in Medicine (in press).

3. Robinson, D.E., Chen, F. and Wilson, L.S.
   Measurement of Velocity of Propagation from
   Ultrasonic Pulse-Echo Data. Ultrasound in Medicine
   and Biology (in press).

4. Bamber, J.C. and Hill, C.R. Acoustic Properties of
   Normal and Cancerous Human Liver - II Dependence on
   Tissue Structure. Ultrasound in Medicine and
   Biology, 7, 135-144, 1981.

# ULTRASONIC TISSUE DIFFERENTIATION FOR TUMOR DIAGNOSIS

J.M. Thijssen

*Department of Ophthalmology, Sint Radboudziekenhuis, University of Nijmegen, 6500 HB Nijmegen, The Netherlands*

## INTRODUCTION

In many medical disciplines when talking about ultrasonic tissue differentiation people start asking <u>questions</u> like:
Which kind of equipment do I have to buy?
What type of computer do I have to buy?
In ophthalmology, however, one may consider the reverse situation to be valid, so one should say: the answer is: Tissue characterization is used in clinical routine!
And, no wonder, one will ask how is that possible? The answer to this question is at least threefold:
First: in ophthalmology one has relatively good access to the pathology, both in a clinical sense, which favours unambiguous conclusions about localisation; and in an acoustical sense. So the ultrasound arrives at the structures of interest without much distortion by intervening tissues.
Second: the equipment used, at least in Europe, may be called standardized, because one manufacturer has been producing the similar pieces of equipment for more than 15 years now (Kretztechnik 7200 MA). This implies that much clinical knowledge has been gained by people in many different countries which is now available to anybody who buys this equipment.
Third: a rather simple and sufficient method of calibrating the equipment with a tissue model has been devised (Till 1975) and so the clinical results are repeatable and what is even more important exchangeable between all the different ophthalmologists! It may be quite a surprise to learn that a rather simple A-mode apparatus is concerned. So in conclusion: in ophthalmology a lot of fine clinical work is performed with a standardized and calibrated A-scanner (cf. Ossoinig, 1974, Poujol, 1974, and for a survey Thijssen and Verbeek, 1981). An example of the pictures one may expect in ophthalmological diagnosis is shown in Fig. 1.

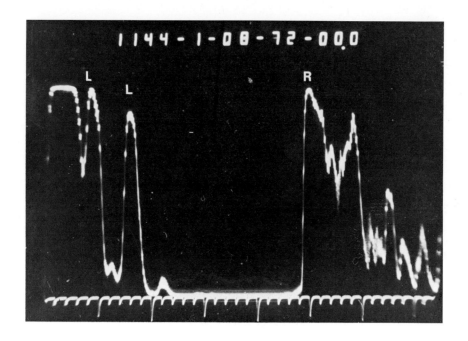

*Figure 1. A-mode echogram of a healthy eye, central appli-
cation on cornea. Lens echoes (L) and retina
peak (R), echolucent vitreous.*

A healthy eye, which is transparent for light, is
also sonolucent. The reflections occur at the transitions
of the various eye media: cornea, lens front and back.
Furthermore echoes are caused by the retina and further
layers of the eyeball and finally from the contents of
the orbit, such as: fat tissue, muscles and optic nerve.
It should be mentioned that in diagnosis the application
of the transducer is generally at the conjunctiva instead
of at the cornea as is the case in Fig. 1. The anterior
(left) part of the echogram is more simple than as is
shown in Fig. 2.

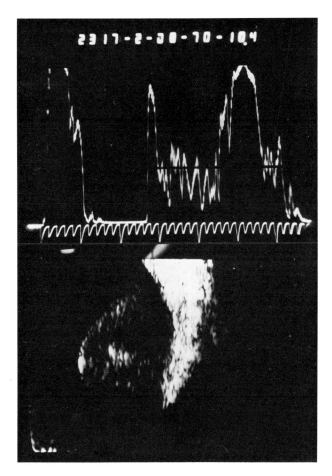

*Figure 2. A- and B-mode echograms of an eye containing a melanoma of the choroid. Note medium reflectivity and regular texture of tumour echoes (T).*

Here we see an eye containing a huge mass behind a strongly prominant retina. The A-mode echogram was obtained while hitting the tumour perpendicularly, which shows up from the high retinal peak. The tumour mass is characterized by a rather homogeneous and medium to low reflective pattern, with low attenuation. These, so-called quantitative, criteria apply to a melanoma but also to a subretinal hemorrhage, which is quite a problem. By contrast, the subretinal tumour in Fig. 3 is highly reflective and regular. These characteristics cannot be seen in the upper echogram, at normal equipment sensitivity, but only at reduced sensitivity, as shown in the lower echogram. The pattern is indicative of a hemangioma.

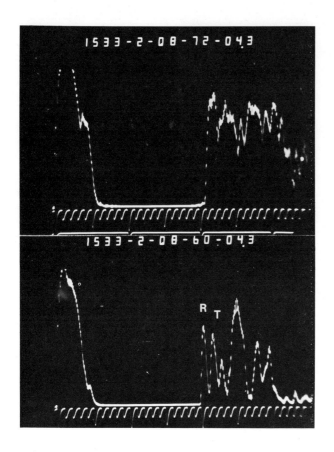

*Figure 3. Upper trace: Echogram from suspected region, note apparent shortening of eye length. Lower trace: 12 dB lowered sensitivity. Tumour echoes (T) now visible behind detached retina (R).*

One should be aware, however, that the quantitative criteria mentioned above are to be complemented by other criteria:

Kinetic criteria are to be found in the mobility of structures, like aftermovements and in the motility of structures as is often observed in malignant tumours (neovascularisation).

Anatomical criteria, most often obtained from B-mode echograms apply to the pathognomonic shape of some tumours and to the localisation of these tumours.

The most important quantitative criteria are listed below: the reflectivity level, which is the size of the echoes at the A-mode screen. It should be repeated: this is a useful criterion only when a calibrated apparatus is used!

the attenuation: which is the rate of decrease of the echo amplitude in the tissue

the texture: which is the distribution of the

echoes and their amplitude in the pathological region, and which is most clearly demonstrated in a histogram.

The tissue characterization discussed so far is no more than a probability that one of the considered alternatives is actually the kind of tumour we will find after histological examination. This means that: although, a relatively high level of differential diagnosis is possible in echo ophthalmology, computer analysis of echograms would still be the most helpful in improving tissue characterization.

This paper will present the A-mode video analysis as performed in the Biophysics Laboratory, then the approach to B-mode video analysis is discussed and finally a few kinds of analysis of the radiofrequency echograms are presented.

ANALYSIS OF VIDEO ECHOGRAMS

By accurately performing measurements through the computer programs one may expect to repeat the clinical diagnosis in the first place and to improve the reliability in the second place. For that purpose the amplitude level of the echoes, the attenuation of the ultrasound, the texture of the echograms which is expressed by the amplitude histogram, and if necessary, the relative reflectivity level of a selected echo are estimated.

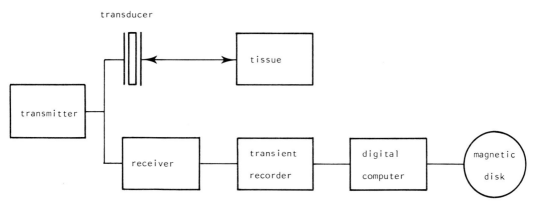

Figure 4. Block diagram of data acquisition equipment for on-line processing of A-mode echograms (Thijssen et al. 1981[a]).

The equipment consists of a normal A-mode apparatus
(Kretztechnik 7200 MA) which is connected to a transient
recorder (Fig. 4). This device collects an echogram in a
digital memory. The acquisition is triggered by taking a
photograph with a Polaroid camera at the A-mode apparatus.
The transient recorder transfers the stored echogram on a
command into the computer memory and the computer commands
the recorder to store the next echogram. This cycle is
repeated quickly and after 24 echograms have been collected the computer starts the analysis. The results of this
analysis are displayed in the examination room on a monitor screen of the computer terminal.

The first stage in the data analysis is the quality
control. Because some time is needed to store 24 echograms
(3 seconds) it is conceivable that the data are disturbed
by unwanted movements of the transducer with respect to
the eye of the patient. The examiner gets a quasi-3 dimensional display of the A-mode echograms (Fig. 5).

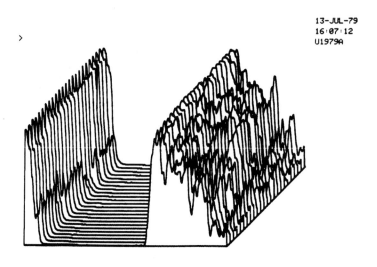

13-JUL-79
16:07:12
U1979A

Figure 5. Isometric display of stored echograms may be
used for control of data acquisition (Thijssen
et al. 1981$^a$).

The advantages of collecting 24 echograms are that
this procedure enables a statistical analysis, because
one may expect that the echograms are slightly different,
and further that by slight movements the pathological
tissue is screened over a considerable volume and not
along a single echographic trace. Another point to re-
mark is that by storing the gain characteristic curve
of the echographic equipment into the computer we are

able to correct each individual echopeak for the non-linear gain compression in the equipment (cf. Kervel and Thijssen, 1980, Thijssen and Kervel, 1981). So we get the echoamplitudes on a true decibel scale.

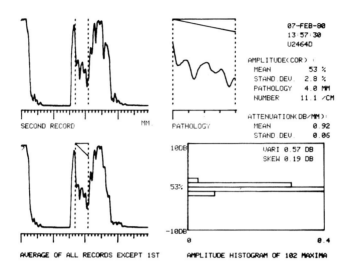

*Figure 6. Output of the analysis program in the case of a melanoma (Thijssen et al. 1981$^a$). For details see text.*

Figure 6 shows as an example a melanoma of the choroid. The upper part is a single echogram, with the vertical lines indicating the tumour, just behind the retina. The lower left picture is the average of 24 echograms. The region of interest is shown in expanded way in the upper right part. The oblique line on top of it displays the regression line through the peaks and it is an estimate of the attenuation within the tissue. The value of the attenuation is given to the right of the picture and it appears to be 0.92 dB/mm. As can be seen the reflectivity level is given in % of the maximum display height (after correction of the attenuation) which is a meaningful figure since we are using a <u>calibrated</u> A-mode equipment. The final picture, bottom <u>right</u> is a 90° rotated amplitude histogram which is unimodal and narrow. We have applied this kind of analysis to the diagnosis of melanoma and objectively documented the differentiation from other kinds of intra ocular tumours. The application to intraorbital tumours seems very promising, but our study is not finished at present.

The analysis of B-mode pictures started in our laboratory recently and only a few preliminary results will be discussed. A major advantage of analysing B-mode instead of A-mode echograms is the opportunity for investigating a particular tissue volume systematically. The goals of processing B-mode echograms by a computer may be divided in: improvement of the structural information, that is better display of the anatomy and of pathological structures and secondly: analysis of tissue texture, whether or not in an automatic classification and decision scheme. It will be clear that the first goal serves the visual evaluation of the echograms by the doctor, while the second one may be considered as an important step towards what is often called "computer diagnosis".

The image processing algorithms may be divided into gray scale manipulations (contrast improvement) and spatial filtering (improvement of resolution and contour enhancement). The texture analysis comprises: gray scale statistics, and $1^{st}$ and $2^{nd}$ order spatial statistics. The various techniques will now be illustrated with an echogram from a metastatic tumour in the liver.

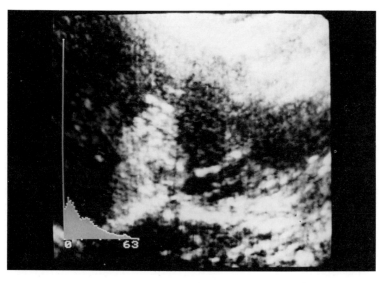

Figure 7. Longitudinal scan through liver containing a
        metastasis. Gray level histogram superimposed.

Figure 7 displays the original picture, digitized and stored in the computer memory and reproduced with a 64 gray level scan converter on a TV monitor. It shows a longitudinal scan through the liver, with the diaphragm left below in the picture, the gray scale histogram is depicted over the echogram. Figure 8 shows the same picture after gray scale manipulation: the gray scale histogram is stretched over the range from 0 to 40 of the original picture, resulting in an improved contrast of the lower gray scale levels (non-specular reflections in the tissue).

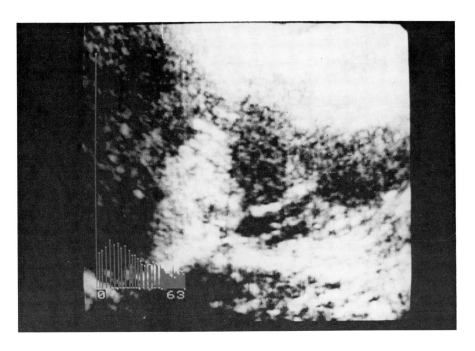

*Figure 8. Picture of Fig. 7 after stretching of lower part of histogram.*

An example of spatial filtering is shown in Fig. 9: the region of interest is high pass filtered by a spatial deconvolution algorithm and a great improvement of the lateral resolution resulted. The gain in image quality is not obvious because no anatomical structure is present in the analysed region. The right slide shows the result after homomorphic high pass filtering combined with gray scale manipulations. This kind of display is optimally suited to texture analysis but obviously not at all to visual evaluation!

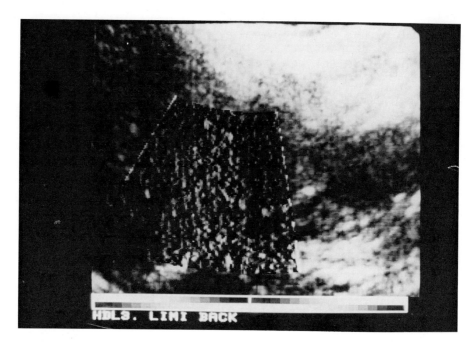

*Figure 9. Result of spatial high pass filtering of suspec-
ted region. Note coarsening of texture caused
by lateral "sharpening".*

One has to decide what the goal is before selecting
the kind of image processing. In this field "the sky is
the limit" and a task in the near future will be to se-
lect the meaningful algorithms and then to achieve clinical experience.

ANALYSIS OF A-MODE RF ECHOGRAMS

So far only video signals have been considered which implies that the echographic "sight" is blurred by the distortion of the signals by the equipment.

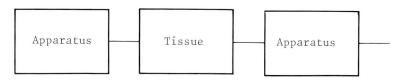

*Figure 10. Definition of problem: removing the influence of the equipment on the echogram.*

This is illustrated with Figure 10, where we can see that the echographic output signal results from the transmitting part of the equipment and after passing through the tissue from the receiving part as well. The first aim of RF analysis may be to remove these influences. But generally the pathological tissue under investigation is inside the body, so we also have distortion by the intervening tissue layers. Two spectral deconvolution methods for getting rid of the distortions and which produce "clean" information about the acoustic properties of the pathology will be discussed now.

A clinical problem which is of relevance is the differentiation of intraocular membranes. In different kinds of pathological conditions the vitreous body becomes optically opaque and the ophthalmologist wants to know whether the retina is detached or not. So the question is to differentiate vitreal membranes from a detached retina, or from a detached choroid.

The implemented computer analysis is called inverse filtering. The potential of this analysis was investigated by applying it to an echo from a flat reflector (Bayer and Thijssen 1981). It was concluded that the inverse filtering improves the axial resolution by a factor of two. This results in a broadening of the bandwidth by a factor of two as well. Additionally, the information about the phase of the echoes is improved, by the symmetry of the echowaveform after inverse filtering, so one gets better information on the transitions in the acoustic impedance at the front and rear surfaces of the membranes.

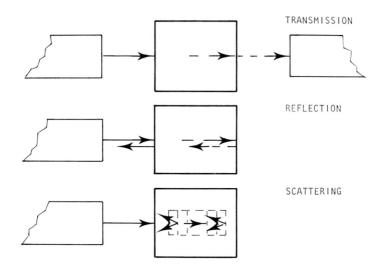

TRANSMISSION

REFLECTION

SCATTERING

*Figure 11. Three methods for estimation of the attenuation coefficient.*

In conclusion: inverse filtering may become a useful tool in the differential diagnosis of intraocular membranes. Futher applications are to be found in impediography, which is a mapping of the acoustic impedances of the various tissues.

The last subject that will be discussed is the in vivo estimation of the attenuation of ultrasound and its dispersion, which is commonly called the attenuation frequency slope. Various methods of measurement have been described in literature. In Fig. 11, upper trace, we see a transmission measurement that is not usable in most diagnostic applications. The middle sketch shows a method in which the specular reflections of the front and back surfaces of the pathology are used to estimate the attenuation, a method not conceivable to use in in vivo applications. The lower picture shows the method of choice: the backscattered ultrasound energy from various parts of the pathological tissue is used.

The received echogram, and, therefore, the tissue volume under investigation, is devided in small parts. Repetition of this measurement at several lateral positions will improve the reliability of the estimate of the attenuation slope, because a larger tissue volume is considered. Inhomogeneity and anisotropy of the tissue are thus removed from the results. The next step in the procedure is to calculate the spectra of all the various small volumes as defined and taking the average at all the depths over the different lateral positions.

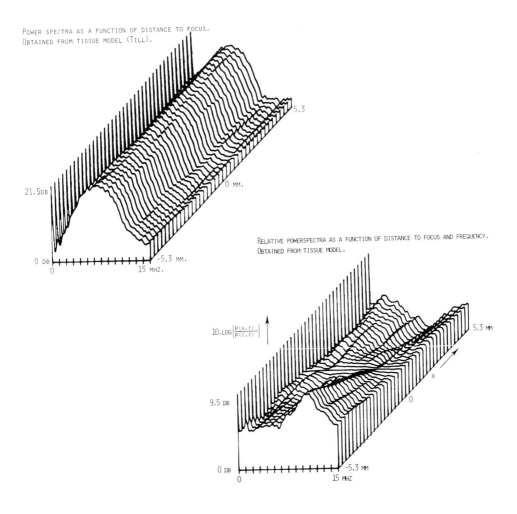

Figure 12. Left: Spectrogram from 30 mm tissue phantom.
Right: Same data after normalization to central spectrum. Note the clear decrease of
energy at high frequencies with increasing
depth (Thijssen et al. 1981[b]).

In Fig. 12 left in the 3D display of the spectra as
a function of depth in the tissue is shown (cf. Thijssen
et al. 1981). Although the frequencies in the figure
range from 0-15 MHz, it must be stated that the meaningful data are between 3 and 11 MHz. The right picture displays the same data, but now the spectra are calculated
relative to the spectrum at depth point zero. It is now
quite clear that the more the sound has travelled through
the tissue, the more the high frequencies are suppressed.
This observation is known as positive dispersion of the
attenuation.

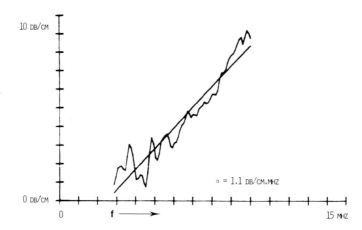

ATTENUATION AS FUNCTION OF FREQUENCY. OBTAINED FROM TISSUE MODEL

$\alpha = 1.1$ DB/CM.MHZ

*Figure 13. Plot of attenuation vs frequency for the data in Figs. 11 and 12. Linear regression yields 1.1 dB/cm MHz (Thijssen et al. 1981<sup>b</sup>).*

In Fig. 13 the attenuation observed in the former pictures is plotted against frequency and the regression line through the data displays the attenuation slope one has been looking for. In this case, which is a tissue phantom, the slope appears to be 1.1 dB/cm MHz. The feasibility of the method to estimate the attenuation slope is herewith demonstrated (cf. Thijssen et al. 1981) and future activities will be devoted to develop the means to apply this method to in vivo tumour diagnosis. At least one group (cf. Lizzi et al. 1981) has devised such a system for ophthalmological diagnosis. The activities of the Biophysics Laboratory will be directed to achieve a combination of real time B-mode display and on-line-A-, or even B-mode RF echogram analysis by a digital computer.

ACKNOWLEDGEMENTS

The author thanks H. van Dooren, R. Kruizinga, A. Bayer and M. Cloostermans for their contributions to this work. The research has been supported by The Health Organization TNO, and the Queen Wilhelmina Foundation.

REFERENCES

1.  Kervel, S.J.H. and Thijssen, J.M. (1980) A device for the display and adjustment of the non-linear gain curve of ultrasonic A-mode equipment. Ultrasonics 19: 40-42.

2. Lizzi, F.L., Coleman, D.J., Feleppa, E., Herbst, J., and Jaremko, N. Digital processing and imaging modes for clinical ultrasound. In: "Ultrasonography in Ophthalmology". Eds. J.M. Thijssen, and A.M. Verbeek. Junk, Publ., Den Haag. Pp. 405-410.

3. Ossoinig, K.C. (1974) Quantitative echography - the basis of tissue differentiation. J. Clin. Ultras. 2: 33-46.

4. Poujol, J. (1974) Echographic diagnosis of tumors in ophthalmology. In: "Ultrasonics in Medicine". Eds. M. de Vlieger, D.N. White and V.R. McCready. Exc. Medica, Amsterdam. Pp. 147-165.

5. Thijssen, J.M., Bayer, A.L., and Cloostermans, M.J. T.M. (1981[a]). Computer assisted echography: statistical analysis of A-mode video echograms obtained by tissue sampling. Med. Biol. Eng. & Comput. 19: 437-442.

6. Thijssen, J.M., Cloostermans, M.J.T.M. and Bayer, A.L. (1981[b]). Measurement of ultrasound attenuation in tissues from scattered reflections: in-vitro assessment of applicability. In: "Ultrasonography in Ophthalmology" Eds. J.M. Thijssen, A.M. Verbeek. Junk. Publ., Den Haag. Pp. 431-439.

7. Thijssen, J.M. and Kervel, S.J.H. van (1981) Electronic tissue model. In: "Ultrasonography in Ophthalmology". Eds. J.M. Thijssen and A.M. Verbeek. Junk Publ., Den Haag. Pp. 527-530.

8. Thijssen, J.M., and Verbeek, A.M. (1981). Computer analysis of A-mode echograms from choroidal melanoma. In: "Ultrasonography in Ophthalmology". Eds. J.M. Thijssen, and A.M. Verbeek. Junk, Publ. Den Haag. Pp. 123-129.

# RHYTHMIC SONOGRAPHIC PALPATION (ECHOSISMOGRAPHY). A NEW TECHNIQUE FOR MALIGNANT, BENIGN TUMOR DIFFERENTIATION BY A SONOGRAPHIC APPROACH OF TUMOR ELASTICITY

A. Eisenscher, G. Pelletier and Ph. Jacquemard

*Centre Hospitalier Paul-Morel, Vesoul, France*

## SUMMARY

A new method to characterize tissues through the studying of the elasticity has been developped.
After the shaking of the organ to be studied some sinusoïdal waves have been recorded in the time motion mode and analysed.

## INTRODUCTION

Though classical palpation, malignant tumors are characterized by beeing hard, indeformable, and adherent to surrounding tissues. They have lost the elasticity characterizing normal tissues.
Classical ultrasonographic investigations only give morphological information, they are unable to appreciate tissue elasticity, where as a physical examination is.
Since superficial tumors only are palpable, physical investigation is limited in deepth-exploration.
The analyzing of elastic waves propagation in human tissues enables indirect palpation in deepth. This analysis is done either in real-time echoscopy or more accurately, in time motion.

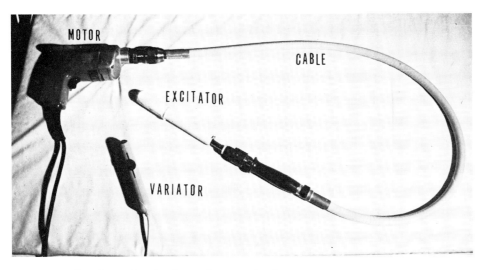

Figure 1 (a-b) Mechanical excitator device
The amplitude of the signal depends from the angle.
Rotation speed can be choosed by means of an electrical va-
riator.

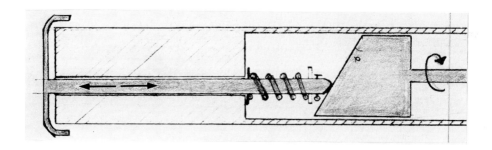

THEORETICAL CONSIDERATIONS

A) Oscillatory system behaviour

In the case of organic tissues only aperiodic wave motion can be considered. Thenfore we have to provoke and maintain the oscillations. This enables the phenomena to be spread in time.

We use entertained oscillations by imposing a rythmic motion to the system, by meens of a mechanical excitator. (Fig 1)

The target organ then becomes a resonator, which is the place for forced oscilations, inducted by the excitator.

The response of the resonating surroundings at the excitation, concerning the amplitude, and the shape of elastic waves is different according to the nature of tissues. (sane, tumoral benign or malignant ones)

For forced oscillations, the reponse in amplitude of elastic wave propagation is function of frequency range and of the regularity of the excitation signal.

Frequency range : For an equal excitation intensity the response in amplitude of the resonating tissue can be different, according to the frequency we use.

We found that the optimal excitation frequency is about 1 excitation every second.

B) Application of theoretical elements

a) Excitation of a benign tumor :

When considering a benign tumor as well differenciated, we can suppose that this tumor is relatively independant from its surroundings.This particularity makes it freer and more accessible to forced oscillations by choosing the suitable excitations.

b) Excitation of a malignant tumor :

When a tumor is adhe ent and invasive, its structure is modified this kind of tumor is not clearly delimited from the surrounding tissues.

The normal tissue-tumor relation becomes closer therefore it introduces a discontinuity in elastic behavior.

Under mechanical excitation, the unit "tumor-sane tissue" responds to the excitation by: - a loose of defined limits
- an increased resistance to forced oscillations
- no oscillatory response under a defined excitation level

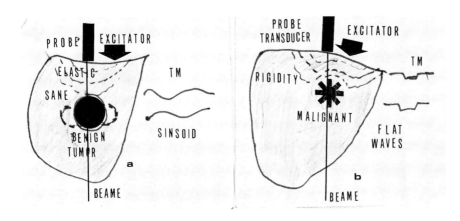

Figure 2
a) Response of normal tissues after excitation : sinusoïdal
type curve. Deformable benign tumor
b) Response of tumoral tissues at excitation of a frequency of
1 pulsation per second, and an applied pression of 500 gr on
4 cm2 : flat type curve because of the rigidity and adhesitivy
of malignants tumors.

The fact that a defined excitation level in amplitude exists in
malignant tumors sems to explain the flattening of the curves
obtained in this type of tumors ( schema b)
Benign tumors have more motion  liberty in surrounting tissues
because (schema a)


  C) Remarks
    The differential diagnostic between benign and malignant tumor
is accurate if exploration conditions are satisfactory :
- a thin abdominal wall, - possibility of applying excitations as
near as possible to the lesion.
Some malignant tumors may give benign type oscillations if then
are small and pourly adherent.
The application of too strong excitation forces, higher than the
excitation level may give pseudo-elastic waves.


MATERIAL AND METHOD

    When  displayed in classical sonographic technique the lesion
is located with calipers.
Calipers allow the recognizing of the tumor level at any moment in
time motion mode.
Vibrations are then applied on the skin as near as possible to the
lesion. A regular frequency of one impulsin per second at a constant
pressure of 500 gr on 4 cm2 is used. (Fig 3)
The response of resonating tissues to vibratory excitation is recorded and characterized by the amplitude of the oscillations (sinusoïdal shape)

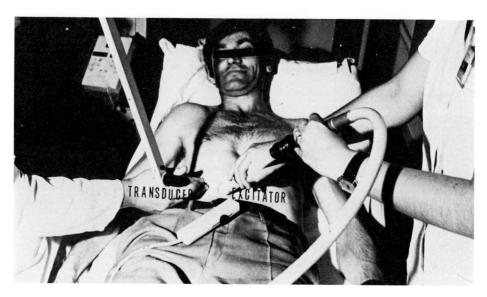

Figure 3  Examination technique

- For sane tissues and benign tumors located between 2 and 10 cm deepth, the average oscillatory amplitude is 0,5 cm when the technical conditions mentionned above are used. This oscillation amplitude is mesured on the sinusoïdal waves recorded in time motion mode.

- For malignant tissues, under a pression of 1 kg on 4 cm2, the response in oscillatory amplitude is weak, there fore flat wave are obtained in TM.
It is also possible to record and analyze the oscillatory amplitude in realtime mode using the magnetic tape.

CASES :

At the begining we studied 133 tumors, using manual vibratory excitation.
Since May 1981, we have built a mechanical vibratory device (Fig 1 and 3)
It gives regular reproductible oscillations with a frequency of oscillation/second and an amplitude of 1,5 cm.
72 tumors displayed in B mode sonography were studied and temporary classified benign or malignant as in conventional investigation.
We completed then the examination by the echosismographic rythmic palpation method. The results were compared with those of classical sonography.
50 tumors (from 72) could be studied by this method.
22 tumors could not be studied in echosismography because the were located deeper than 10 CM from the skin or hided by ribs. The size of the masses was ranged from 0,5 cm for the smallest one to 13 cm for the biggest one. The studied tumors were located in the :
liver (23) , kidney (21), breast (18), pancreas (8) gallblader (2).

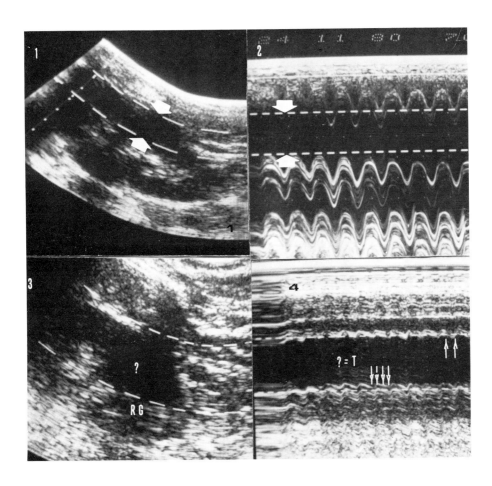

Figure 4

1) B Mode sonography of a kidney, cyst, display, localisation of lesion by calipers (a ows)

2) Elastic oscillations of this benign lesion

3) Sonolucent kidney lesion not characteristic in B mode sonography

4) Flat type oscillations and rigidity in echo-sismographie, malignant type
   Histologicaly prooved nephroblastoma

RESULTS   (see table)

        Echosismography could be perfⱴrmed in 70 % of  the sonographi-
caly visualised tumors.
- The sensivity was 69,5 %
- THE specificity  100   %

| | Benign 31 | | | Malignant 19 | | |
|---|---|---|---|---|---|---|
| Typical echosismographic oscillations | 31 | 100 | % | 16 | 84,2 | % |
| Echosismographic errors | 0 | 0 | % | 3 | 15,8 | % |
| Accurate diagnostic in B mode or real time US | 26 | 87,8 | % | 12 | 63 | % |
| Error diagnostic in B mode out realtime sonography | 5 | 16,2 | % | 7 | 36,9 | % |
| Diagnostic benefits of echosismography compared to classical sonography | 5 | 16,2 | % | 4 | 25 | % |

| Examnated tumors | | Echosismography possible | | Echosismography impossible | | Error Dg. in sismogra. |
|---|---|---|---|---|---|---|
| LIVER | 23 | 17 | 74 % | 6 | 26 % | 1 |
| KIDNEY | 21 | 13 | 62 % | 8 | 38 % | 1 |
| BREASTS | 18 | 12 | 66 % | 6 | 33,4% | 1 |
| PANCREAS | 8 | 6 | 75 % | 2 | 25 % | 0 |
| GALBLADDER | 2 | 2 | 100 % | 0 | 0 % | 0 |
| TOTAL CASES | 72 | 50 | 70 % | 22 | 18 % | 3 |

TABLE  OF  RESULTS

DISCUSSION (Fig 5 and 6)
        Benign tumors always gave sinusoïdal type oscillations. Most of
this kind of tumors were semi-liquid or solid.
Malignant tumors gave typical flat curves in 84 % cases.
Some malignant tumors (16 %) gave benign type sinusoïdal oscillations
They had a small size, less then 2 cm diamenter. Some of them where
to superficial so they had easily induced oscillations over the
excitation level.

42

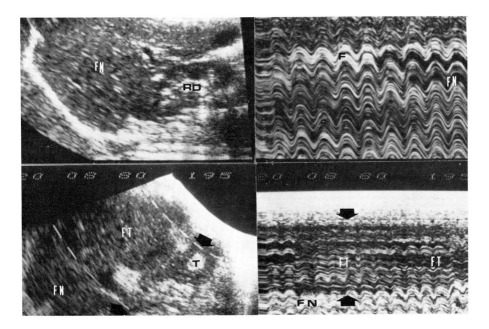

Figure 5
1) Normal liver : (F) 2. Sinusoïdal type waves in sane tissue.
3 Tumoral liver (T) 4. Flat waves typical of malignacy.

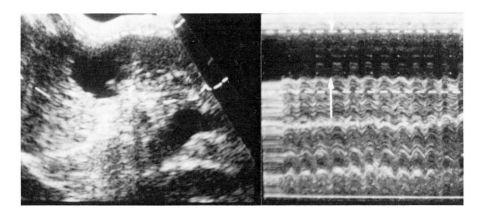

Figure 6
1) Liquid collection in liver, it is difficult to classify this
lesion in B mode sonography

2) Typical malignant lesion (Histologicaly confirmted necrotic
metastasis.

CONCLUSION

Echosismography introduces in sonography the possibility of objective palpation by the study of tissue elasticity.
It is easy to perform with classical sonographic equipement, TM mode or real time magnetic tape recording. The mechanical excitator device is also easy to build.
In order to improve our technique we are trying to treat our results with a computer. The reaction of on oscillating tissulary system at an excitation can be studed by Fouriers transformations.
The results we have obtained seem to be reliable, with 47 accurate diagnostics out of 50 investigated tumors.

BIBLIOGRAPHY

1) EISENSCHER A. Echosismographie.
   Nouvelle Méthode pour différencier les processus bénins de for-mation malignes par l´étude ultrasonore complémentaire de l'élasticité des tumeurs.

   Congrés National de la S.F.A.U.M.B. ROUEN 25, 26, 27 Septembre 1980

2) DIEULESAINT E. et ROYER D.
   Ondes élastiques dans les solides.
   Editions MASSON 1974

3) EISENSCHER A.
   Echosismography - A new method for tissu caracterisation by echographic palpation and tumor elasticity display under rythmic compression.
   4 th European Congres on Ultrasonic in Medecine. May 17 - 24 1981
   Abstract 33, page 14, Excerpta medica ED.

KEY WORDS

- Palpation, sonography
- Tissue characterisation
- TM

# ASPIRATION OF 100 SOLID MASSES UNDER ULTRASONIC GUIDANCE

M. Afschrift[1], P. Nachtegaele[1], D. Voet[1], J.L. De Loof[1], J. Hamers[2] and W. Van Hove[2]

[1]*Department of Internal Medicine and Echography and* [2]*Department of Haematology, Akademisch Ziekenhuis, Ghent, Belgium*

ABSTRACT

Fine needle aspirations were performed in 100 echogenic masses under real-time ultrasonic guidance. In 93 cases there was only one needle pass. Seventy seven malignant masses were punctured. In 67 of the samples, malignant cells could be detected; 6 samples were suspect of malignancy while 4 were not. Two out of 12 benign lesions were cytologically suspect of malignancy (one renal adenoma and one hypertrophic renal column). In 11 liver nodules no definite diagnosis could be reached, cytology showing only atypia of liver cells. Benign masses may be included in this group. In this series no complications occurred. These results confirm the usefulness of ultrasonically guided aspirations.

INTRODUCTION

Solid tumors present on sonograms as echogenic masses. Reflectivity may vary considerably : some tumors are highly echogenic, while others give rise to low intensity echoes. Sometimes reflectivity is so poor that fluid collections may be simulated. Rarely solid masses may even be partially or entirely echofree, due to fluid secretion or to necrosis. Echogenicity may even vary among different metastatic nodules of one tumor. In most cases sonographic features are not typical. Even benign masses cannot be differentiated from malignant tumors.

The most direct approach to diagnosis is to perform aspirations under ultrasonic guidance to obtain a tissue specimen for cytologic examination.

In this report, results are presented of ultrasonically guided aspirations of 100 echogenic nodules.

MATERIALS AND METHODS

One hundred echogenic areas were aspirated in 99 patients. In most cases, punctures were done to confirm malignancy or to document tumor spreading. The diameter of the masses ranged from 1 to 10 cm and the depth of the puncture varied from 1 to 9.5 cm. Guidance was performed under real-time ultrasonic control (5 MHz linear-array transducer with central canal, ADR-Kranzbühler). In all cases a fine needle (outer diameter .6 mm) was used, which was introduced through a guide needle. The depth of the puncture was determined on the

TABLE 1. Distribution of aspiration biopsies of solid lesions.

| | | | |
|---|---|---|---|
| LIVER | MALIGNANT TUMORS | | 24 | |
| |   – Hepatocarcinoma | 1 | | |
| |   – Malignant histiocytosis | 1 | | |
| |   – Myeloma | 1 | | |
| |   – Metastatic nodules | 21 | | |
| | NODULES OF UNDETERMINED ORIGIN | | 11 | 35 |
| KIDNEY | MALIGNANT TUMORS | | 14 | |
| |   – Carcinoma | 13 | | |
| |   – Malignant histiocytosis | 1 | | |
| | BENIGN LESIONS | | 2 | |
| |   – Adenoma | 1 | | |
| |   – Hypertrophic column | 1 | | 16 |
| THORAX | MALIGNANT THYMOMA | | 4 | |
| | MALIGNANT LYMPHOMA | | 3 | |
| | MALIGNANT SCHWANNOMA | | 1 | |
| | BRONCHIAL CARCINOMA | | 3 | |
| | PULMONARY LEUKEMIC INFILTRATION | | 1 | |
| | PLEURAL METASTASIS | | 1 | |
| | PLEURAL THICKENING | | 1 | 14 |
| RETROPERITONEAL AREA | MALIGNANT LYMPH NODES | | 6 | |
| | ADRENAL METASTASIS | | 3 | 9 |
| PANCREAS | CARCINOMA | | 6 | |
| | CHRONIC PANCREATITIS | | 1 | 7 |
| NECK | THYROID NODULE | | 3 | |
| | LYMPH NODES | | 4 | |
| |   – Carcinoma | 2 | | |
| |   – Malignant lymphoma | 1 | | |
| |   – TBC | 1 | | |
| | GRANULOMA | | 1 | 8 |
| GENERAL ABDOMINAL AREA | COLON CARCINOMA | | 3 | |
| | CARCINOMA OF UNKNOWN ORIGIN | | 1 | |
| | MALIGNANT LYMPHOMA | | 1 | |
| | LEIOMYOSARCOMA | | 2 | |
| | LEIOMYOMA | | 1 | 8 |
| SPLEEN | MALIGNANT LYMPHOMA | | 1 | |
| | NO MALIGNANT SPLENOMEGALY | | 2 | 3 |
| | | TOTAL | | 100 |

screen of a TV-monitor, because in most cases the needle tip could
not be accurately located during the procedure. When the needle
reached the target area, suction was applied by a 10 ml syringe
while the needle was quickly moved backwards and forwards for four
times. After withdrawing the needle, the tissue specimen was smeared
on glass slides, air dried and stained according to May-Grünwald-
Giemsa. In 93 cases, there was only one needle pass; in 7 a second
aspiration was performed during the same session because the sample
was judged as insufficient. No topical anaesthesia was used. Prior
to each puncture a screening for bleeding and clotting disorders was
performed.

RESULTS

The localizations of the 100 echogenic lesions are specified
in table 1.
Twelve benign lesions were punctured. Two aspirations of kidney
lesions were cytologically suspect of malignancy, which was not confirmed at surgery. The first patient presented with a renal tumor.
Cytologic examination of the aspirated tissue specimen suggested a
well-differentiated carcinoma, but the pathologist classified the
tumor as renal adenoma. The second patient presented with an echogenic area within the right kidney. Intravenous urography suggested a
hypertrophic column. A fine needle aspiration into this region
yielded a sample suspect of malignancy. Nephrotomy did not reveal a
malignant mass. Until now no further information about the clinical
course of these patients is available.
In 11 liver nodules cytology showed only atypia of liver cells.
So far no definite diagnosis has been reached in these cases.
Seventy seven focal areas, ultimately proved to be of malignant origin, were aspirated (Table 2). In 67 (87 %) malignant cells
could be demonstrated in the samples. In 6 cases there was suspicion
of malignancy, while 4 were negative.

DISCUSSION

Solid benign and malignant masses are easily demonstrated by
ultrasound as echogenic areas. However, ultrasonic features are most
often atypical, necessitating further diagnostic investigations.
Therefore fine needle aspirations under ultrasonic guidance may be of
great value to obtain tissue samples for cytologic diagnosis (1, 2,
4-6).
Real-time ultrasonic guidance is a very attractive method to
that purpose. The needle can easily be guided through the central
canal of the transducer. The target area can also continuously be
monitored during the puncture, while in some cases even the needle
tip penetrating the mass can be visualized. In our series even small
solid masses were successfully aspirated, even when situated in
retroperitoneal organs.
To minimize the risks, in most cases only one aspiration was
performed. Moreover liver nodules were not aspirated if they were
situated just beneath the liver capsule. Some hypervascular echogenic tumors, such as adenomas or haemangiomas might indeed cause

TABLE 2. Cytologic diagnosis of focal malignant lesions.

| | Nr | Malignancy | Suspicion of malignancy | No malignancy |
|---|---|---|---|---|
| LIVER | 24 | 20 | 2 | 2 |
| PANCREAS | 6 | 4 | 2 | – |
| KIDNEY | 14 | 12 | 1 | 1 |
| RETROPERITONEAL AREA | 9 | 8 | – | 1 |
| ABDOMINAL AREA | 7 | 6 | 1 | – |
| THORAX | 13 | 13 | – | – |
| NECK | 3 | 3 | – | – |
| SPLEEN | 1 | 1 | – | – |
| | 77 | 67 (87 %) | 6 | 4 |

severe bleeding after puncturing.

Seventy seven masses were aspirated which subsequently proved
to be of malignant origin. Although in the vast majority only one
aspiration was performed, malignant cells were demonstrated in a
very high percentage of the samples. This seems to indicate that
multiple aspirations in various directions into a tumor are not
necessary. The risk of bleeding and of spreading of tumor cells may
thus be lowered.

Specimens from 11 out of 35 liver nodules did not yield evidence of malignancy. It is interesting to emphasize that 6 of these
nodules were strongly echogenic, which features may also be observed
in haemangiomas. Although false negative results are probably included in this group, some of them might indeed represent benign
masses. As to the two kidney lesions with a possibly false cytological suspicion of malignancy, we have to point first to the well
known problem of differential diagnosis between renal adenoma and
well-differentiated adenocarcinoma (8), and secondly to the lack of
follow-up of these cases.

Despite the absence of local anaesthesia, patients only com-
plained of minimal discomfort, even when deep seated lesions were
punctured. There were no bleeding episodes. Although in most patients
the follow-up was too limited to judge about an eventually needle
tract seeding of malignant cells, we certainly did not have evidence
of it; anyhow other reports indicate that needle tract growth of
tumor is very rarely observed with fine needle aspirations (3, 7).

CONCLUSION

The results of this series confirm the high usefulness of ultrasonic guidance of punctures. By this method tissue samples for cytologic examination may be obtained, without major discomfort to patients and at a low complication rate. Cytology offers a quick and reliable diagnostic assessment for solid echogenic nodules.

REFERENCES

1. Chandrasekhar, A.J., Reynes, C.J. and Churchill, R.J. (1976) : Chest, 70, 627.
2. Hancke, S., Holm, H.H. and Kock, F. (1975) : Surg. Gynecol. Obstet., 140, 361.
3. Holm, H.H., Pedersen, J.F., Kristensen, J.K., Rasmussen, S.N., Hancke, S. and Jensen, F. (1975) : Radiol. Clin. North Amer., 13, 493.
4. Kristensen, J.K., Holm, H.H., Rasmussen, S.N., Barlebo, H. (1972) : Scand. J. Urol. Nephrol., 6 (suppl. 15), 49.
5. Lutz, H., Weidenhiller, S. and Rettenmaier, G. (1973) : Schweiz. Med. Wschr., 103, 1030.
6. Schwerk, W.B. and Schmitz-Moormann, P. (1981) : Cancer, 48, 1469.
7. von Schreeb, T., Arner, O., Skovsted, G. and Wikstad, N. (1967) : Scand. J. Urol. Nephrol., 1, 270.
8. Zajicek, J. (1979) : In : Cytology of infradiafragmatic organs. Aspiration biopsy cytology, part 2, 14. Editor : S. Karger, Basel, München, Paris, London, New York, Sydney.

# THE RESTRICTIONS IMPOSED BY THE ACOUSTIC PROPERTIES OF THE SKULL TO IMAGE CEREBRAL TUMORS WITH ULTRASOUND

D.N. White

*Kingston, Canada*

The first reported attempts to make images from the living human brain with pulse-echo ultrasonic reflection techniques were made in 1950. In their paper to the American Neurological Association, Ballantyne et al. (1950) stated that with their A-mode display 'multiple echoes have been obtained from within the skull' and went on to state that 'the greatest difficulty with this technique arises in interpretation, because multiple echoes are received from various tissue and organ interfaces'. Using the example of the two-dimensional sonar techniques with their PPI display that had been developed during World War II for anti-submarine detection, it appeared only necessary to add the display of a second spatial dimension to the A-mode display of the echoes that were being ranged in order to make sense, with such a B-mode display of these 'multiple echoes'. Howry made such a B-mode spatial display in 1954 (Fig.1) but found the image he obtained so unsatisfactory that sub-

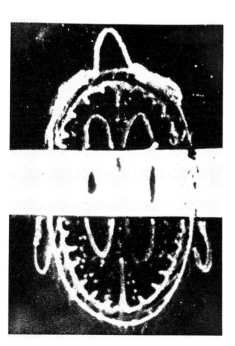

Fig. 1. The first tomogram known to have been made of the brain by Douglass Howry about 1954. The tomogram is in the horizontal plane and comprises the central area of the illustration displaying, presumably, the cerebral midline and ventricular walls on a white background. The black regions were sketched in by hand by Dr. Howry for the reader's orientation.
Published by permission of Ultramedison of Kingston.

sequently he devoted his attention to the imaging of soft tissue regions with much more success. Enthusiasm for this technique waned, especially in the United States, following the pessimistic report of the U.S. Atomic Energy Commission (Moore, 1955). It revived however after Leksell (1956) demonstrated that the A-mode echoencephalographic technique could demonstrate displacement of the cerebral midline structures in unilateral deforming cerebral disease. In the late 1950's a number of investigators, including ourselves, undeterred by Howry's experience, began again to look at the brain with pulse-echo B-mode reflection techniques. By 1962 we had built a primitive sector scanner with which we made our first B-scan of the living human head (Fig. 2). We were dissatisfied with this display which we ascribed to the poor electronics of the system and accordingly, in conjunction with Makow of the National Research Council of Canada developed a much more sophisticated compound circumferential scanning device.

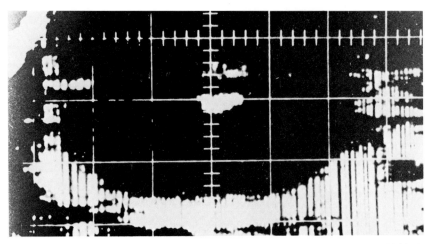

Fig. 2. A horizontal tomogram of the human brain made in 1963 in the author's laboratory with very primitive equipment. The nose is to the right and the occiput to the left. Only portions of the ventricles and falx cerebri are displayed.

At the same time a number of other centres throughout the world were building similar systems. We were disappointed to find, in 1964, that the scanner built by Makow and ourselves produced images of the brain which were only marginally better than those we had obtained with our primitive equipment and which were certainly quite inadequate for diagnostic purposes (Fig. 3). Other workers building scanning systems had the same depressing experience. Belatedly, we came to the conclusion that the difficulties arose not from engineering limitations but as a result of the acoustic properties of the skull and we embarked upon a ten year project of studying these properties (White,

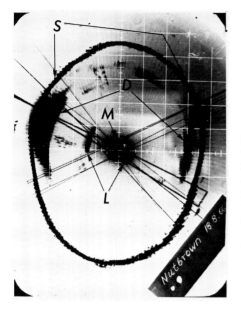

Fig. 3. A horizontal tomogram of the human brain made with the scanner originally developed by Makow and the author in 1964 and later further developed by Makow when this scan was made in 1966. The nose is below and the occiput above. Again only portions of the ventricular system are displayed.

1976, White et al., 1978).

The early history of B-scan echoencephalography with the pulse-echo reflection technique is therefore a classical example of poor scientific technique. Instead of being preceded by basic research work into the physical difficulties that would be encountered in attempts to image the brain by scanning ultrasonic pulses across the brain, we, together with a number of other investigators, were in such a hurry to develop the first clinically useful scanning system that we proceeded directly to build such a system without first adequately researching the acoustic and physical principles involved. In this way millions of dollars and much time were fruitlessly expended.

The fundamental nature of the difficulties imposed by the acoustic properties of the skull only slowly began to be appreciated during the 1970's and was the main reason that the number of papers published on the neurological applications of ultrasound declined after 1968 despite the exponential rise in the number of papers published in other fields of ultrasonic diagnosis (Fig. 4).

## The resolution of spatial images

The quality of the spatial images made of the brain or any other organ will depend both upon the congruity of the display with the objects to be imaged and upon the resolution with which the objects are imaged.

In order to make A-mode images of reflecting interfaces in range the propagation time of a generated ultrasonic pulse and its reflected echo are measured and equated with a given distance in the range dimension. Obviously in order

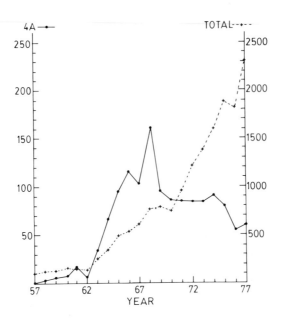

Fig. 4. The total number of papers appearing annually in the world literature since the discovery of midline echoencephalography. The solid line (left hand scale) represents those relating to the neurological application of ultrasound in comparison with the total number of papers relating to all aspects of medical and biological ultrasound (dotted line and right hand scale).

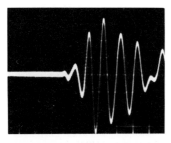

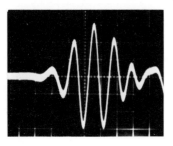

Fig. 5. The electrical pulses generated by an ultrasonic transducer with a rated frequency of 2 MHz and detected by a piezoelectric receiver with a wide frequency bandwidth in the free field (upper) and after propagating through human skull (lower). The amplitudes have been normalised. Each horizontal graticule represents 0.5 µs.

Although passage through the skull has advanced the propagation time of the pulse, caused total attenuation of the pulse (not apparent), differential attenuation of the higher frequencies and increased interference especially in the later cycles of the pulse, the pulse length has been little increased after propagating through the skull.

to display the echoes reflected from interfaces at different depths congruously in range, the velocity of propagation of the different pulses must be known. Ultrasound propagates at different velocities through different tissues and this difference is especially marked when some of these tissues are bony in which the velocity of propagation is approximately twice that in soft tissue. In order to form a two-dimensional B-mode spatial display, it is necessary to scan the ultrasonic beam in the lateral dimension that is being imaged. Under these circumstances the beam will propagate through varying depths of different tissues, in each of which it has a different propagation velocity. As a result the display of the received echoes in range based solely upon their propagation time will be variably incongruous in the range dimension. It can be imagined that if, during the course of a scan, the beam propagated through markedly varying depths of bone this incongruity would become quite marked. Luckily, however, during the course of any B-scan, the relative proportions of the different tissues through which the pulses will propagate does not vary to a marked degree. Under these circumstances, although the range display will not be absolutely congruous with the range of the different reflecting interfaces, the relative incongruity will not be great.

The resolution of the echoes displayed in the range dimension will vary inversely as the length of the pulse detected by the receiving system. It is possible to generate appropriately brief ultrasonic pulses which are stretched to only a minor degree in propagating through soft tissue. The pulses, however, are appreciably prolonged, as will be described, in propagating through the cancellous bone of the diploe of the skull. Nevertheless, the degradation in range resolution that results from this stretching of the ultrasonic pulse is much less than the degradation in resolution in the lateral dimensions imposed by propagation through soft tissues and especially by the skull (Fig. 5).

If it is desired to image also in one of the lateral dimensions as is necessary for any B-mode display, then other factors must be considered. Congruity of the display in either of the two lateral dimensions will depend upon the interfaces from which echoes are received lying in the transducer axis. It is not possible for an imaging system to sense the direction in which the beam propagates but only the direction in which the transducer is orientated. The system will display the echoes received at appropriate ranges as if the reflecting interfaces lay along this sensed axis of the generator receiver. Thus, any factors that cause deflection of the ultrasonic beam, with its maximal intensities of generated energy, from the beam axis along which it normally lies, will result in the echoes reflected by this beam being displayed incongruously in the lateral dimension. Obviously any medium that will cause reflection or refraction of the beam while it is propagating into the tissues to be imaged will result in such incongruity and this

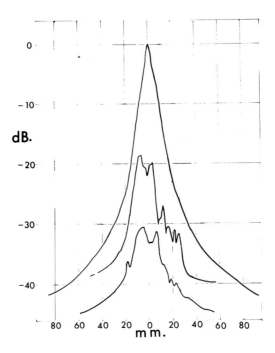

Fig. 6. Intensity distribution curves of the beam generated by a plane faced piston transducer 13 mm in diameter with a nominal frequency of 2 MHz. and measured at the start of the far field where the beam is narrowest. The upper curve is made in the free field and the two lower curves after the beam has propagated through two separate regions of the same human parietal bone being most attenuated in the lowest curve.

If this beam were scanned across point reflecting targets, the receiving system would display the points as lines in the lateral dimension scanned with a width corresponding to the level of sensitivity of the receiving system.

For instance at a receiver sensitivity corresponding to 0 dB a point target in the free field would be displayed as a point but targets returning weaker echoes below this threshold of sensitivity, such as point targets scanned through the skull, would not be displayed. If the receiver sensitivity is increased by 32 dB in order to display point targets scanned through the more attenuating region of the skull (lowest curve) each point target will be displayed twice; one as a horizontal line 10 mm long and 6 mm to the left of its true position and one as a line 3 mm long and 5 mm to the right of its true position. If the same point target was then scanned through the less attenuating portion of the skull and at the same setting of receiver sensitivity, it would be displayed as a horizontal line 36 mm in length.

This degradation of lateral resolution could be reduced if the receiver sensitivity was reduced to 20 dB in which case the point target would appear as two images 5 mm long and 7 mm to the left of its true position and as a point 3 mm to the right of its true position when scanned through the less attenuating regions of the skull (middle curve). It would not be displayed at this level of sensitivity when scanned through the more attenuating region of the skull (lowest curve).

incongruity will increase progressively for structures at increasing range from the reflecting or refracting medium. As will be described, the skull with its markedly different acoustic impedance to that of soft tissue, will be an especially potent medium for causing reflection or refraction of ultrasonic energy incident upon it.

Resolution in either of the two lateral dimensions will vary inversely with the effective beam width. The effective beam width varies with the receiver sensitivity and becomes greater at increasing sensitivity. Ideally resolution would be optimum if the receiver sensitivity was so restricted that the effective beam were infinitely narrow so that reflections from point interfaces would only be displayed by the imaging system as points when the infinitely narrow beam scanned across them. Larger interfaces would likewise be displayed with their correct width and without false enlargement in the lateral dimension being scanned. If it is necessary to increase the dynamic range of the receiving system in order to display echoes of varying intensities, the receiver sensitivity must be increased. This will increase the effective beam width for the echoes of high intensity by an amount equal to the width of the ultrasonic beam corresponding to that level of increased receiver sensitivity. Thus point targets will be displayed as lines in the lateral dimension being scanned of length corresponding to the effective beam width for echoes received at that level of sensitivity above threshold. Line targets will be enlarged by an equal amount. For this reason it is desirable to generate ultrasonic beams that are as narrow as possible throughout a wide dynamic range (Fig. 6, upper curve). While beams of only a few mms in width can readily be generated in the free field, propagation through soft tissues scatters the energy concentrated in the beam to a variable degree with the result that its width increases. This spreading of the beam is especially marked when the ultrasonic pulse propagates through the cancellous bone of the diploe of the skull (Fig. 6, lower curves).

With any ultrasonic reflection technique both the congruity of the display and resolution in the lateral dimensions is poorer in the lateral dimensions than in the range dimension. For these reasons almost all images made with ultrasonic reflection techniques are either in range alone or, if two-dimensional images are desired, combined imaging in range with one of the two lateral dimensions.

## The acoustic properties of the skull

Since they have so much more marked an effect in degrading the images made in the lateral dimension it will be appropriate to discuss the acoustic properties of the skull with reference to imaging in the lateral dimension first, following which the effect of the skull on range resolution becomes readily understood.

It is well known that the skull greatly attenuates the

energy that propagates through it and it is often erroneously believed that this is due to absorption of the energy within the skull. This is not the case and bone absorbs energy no more than other bodily tissues. The gross attenuation of the energy caused by the skull is due to the fact that it is scattered by the skull from its original direction of propagation. This scattering is all the result of the marked impedance mismatch between the skull and soft tissues. As one result, any ultrasonic energy incident upon the outer surface of the skull is reflected backwards to a greater extent than by interfaces between soft tissues. Least energy is reflected backwards when the beam is normally incident upon the skull but an increasing proportion of it is reflected backwards as the angle of incidence increases and indeed, at 27°, the critical angle for soft tissue-bone interfaces, all the energy incident upon the skull is reflected backwards and none can propagate onwards into the bone and underlying brain. For this reason in order to image the underlying brain, it is necessary that the maximal amount of energy propagates through the skull by insuring that it is always incident upon the skull at or near normal incidence. The surface of the skull however is curved except in the temporal areas and it is for this reason that most energy is transmitted into the brain when a scan is performed over the temporal areas and the transducer is kept at, or nearly at, normal incidence. In other areas proportionately more energy is reflected backwards as the transducer scans away from normal incidence and as a result of the curvature of the skull.

Once the energy has coupled into the skull across the

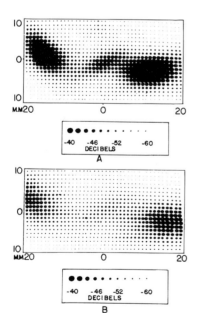

Fig. 7. Intensity distribution plots of energy reflected by a 10 mm sphere of the energy that has propagated through human temporal bone. The sphere reflects back to the generator-receiver energy regardless of its direction of propagation. In the top plot the sphere was 90 mm from the transducer and in the lower plot was 120 mm distant. Two concentrations of energy are clearly seen displaced to either side of the transducer axis in the upper plot. This results from refraction by either side of a crest of bone lying vertically across the transducer axis. The lower plots show that these concentrations of energy are diverging at increasing distances from the transducer.

soft tissue skull interface it is of course subject to other physical processes such as refraction and scattering. The preference for scanning through the temporal area has an unfortunate effect with regard to refraction of the ultrasonic beam. The inner table of the temporal bone is more markedly convoluted than other areas of the skull and these convoluted areas will refract the beam away from its original axis of propagation. A good example of this effect is seen in Figure 7 where the beam has propagated across the temporal bone to intersect a ridge between two convolutional surfaces. As a result, half of the beam has been refracted to the right and the other half to the left and these two refracted portions are diverging as can be seen by the lower plot which is made 3 cms more distant than the other plot. Obviously any interface insonated by either of these two diverging beams and returning an echo detected by the receiving system will be displayed incongruously in the lateral dimensions since the receiving system will perceive it as an echo originating in the transducer axis. It will be noted that the degree of incongruity in the display will increase for echoes originating at greater depths.

These then are the effects of the acoustic mismatch of the skull causing marked backward reflection from its smooth outer surface and refraction of the beam from its convoluted inner surface. However, an equally serious problem arises during the transmission of the energy across the skull as it encounters the cancellous diploe between the outer and inner tables. These diploe approximate in size to the wave-length of the energy being used and therefore will very markedly scatter this energy over wide angles as it couples from the bone into the soft tissues of the diploe and from the soft tissues back into the cancellous bone again and so on. For this reason the energy emerging from the skull is scattered widely and diffusely over a considerable area. Obviously such scattering of the energy normally concentrated around the transducer axis will cause a considerable increase in the beam width (Fig. 6). There will be a consequent degradation of resolution in the lateral dimension. It might be possible, by limiting the dynamic range of the imaging system, to overcome partially this increase in the beam width were it of constant degree. Unfortunately however the pattern of widespread scattering of the beam varies markedly with every small movement of the transducer and its generated beam with respect to the skull (Fig. 8). More importantly the attenuation of the beam will also vary markedly with such movements of the transducer (Fig. 6, two lower curves). Thus, during any scan of the beam across the skull the same interface will return echoes of widely different intensities. When such an echo is received at an intensity just exceeding the threshold for display it will be displayed with optimal resolution in the lateral dimension being scanned. However, if, during the scan, the same interface reflects a more in-

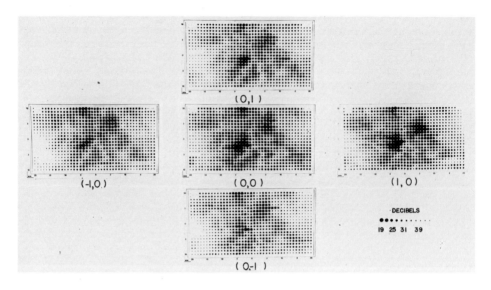

Fig. 8. Five field plots showing the intensity of energy generated by a plane-faced ultrasonic transducer with a rated frequency of 1.5 MHz and made in a plane perpendicular to the beam axis at 200 mm which is twice the distance of the last axial maximum (2P) from the face of the generator.

The plots are made after the energy has made a single passage through the human temporal bone which is moved 1 mm above, below and to left and right of its position for the central plot. The pattern of scattering of the beam by the skull varies greatly with slight movements of the skull relative to the beam.

tense echo much exceeding the threshold for display, the optimal image will have superimposed upon it a larger image with degraded resolution. Such scanning movements of the beam are necessary for imaging in the lateral dimensions with reflection techniques since the beam must be scanned in the corresponding lateral dimension. Hence the pattern of scattering and the degree of widening of the beam will continually be changing during the period of a scan and each accumulated image will be displayed with the worst resolution for that system. It is not usually appreciated how extremely sensitive is this variation in the pattern of scattering of the energy in the beam to the smallest motion of the beam relative to the skull. Figure 9 shows sixteen separate field plots made across the same living head. A holding device was used and every effort was made with each plot to reposition the transducer in exactly the same position as previously. Nevertheless the pattern of the scattered energy varied widely between the plots.

The incongruity of the display in the range dimension due to the increased velocity of propagation through the skull has been mentioned above. If the beam always propa-

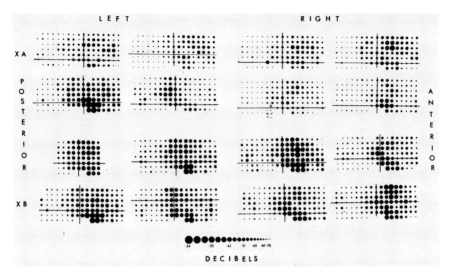

Fig. 9. Field plots of the intensity of ultrasonic energy at 2 MHz transmitted across the same living human head from an unfocussed transducer 13 mm in diameter. The 8 plots on the left were made with the transducer in the left temporal area and vice versa. Each dot is separated from the next dot by 5 mm so that the fields displayed are 8 cms by 3 cms in size. The central axis of the generator is shown by the intersection of the horizontal and vertical lines.

Every effort was made to reposition the transducer in its holding device in exactly the same position for each separate plot. There are nevertheless very great differences in the pattern of the scattered energy from one plot to the next.

gated through the same thickness of skull the <u>relative</u> position of the interfaces displayed in range would show little incongruity. However, as has been pointed out, in order to image in a lateral dimension it is necessary to scan the beam in that lateral dimension. Under these circumstances the beam will propagate through different thicknesses of skull which, in the temporal regions, ranges from 1 mm to 8 mm in width. As a consequence there will be variable degrees of incongruity in the display in range of interfaces imaged with a scanning technique which approximate to the variations in thickness of the skull through which the beam propagates at approximately twice the velocity through soft tissue.

If however the beam is not scanned across the skull but is kept fixed with respect to it, no such varying incongruities in the display result. For this reason it is possible to measure with considerable accuracy and precision, any variations in the range of a single interface resulting from the normal movements of the brain so long as the transducer is kept stationary. Advantage was taken of this fact in measuring the normal pulsations of the brain in range (White, 1981).

Resolution in the range dimension varies inversely with the received pulse length. As mentioned above, in propagating across the cancellous diploe, the energy in the beam is scattered to a marked degree and repeatedly couples from the bone into the soft tissues of the diploe where it propagates at a slower velocity before coupling back into the bone and back into the diploe etc. with appropriately varying velocities of propagation. As a result, in propagating across the cancellous diploe, the pulse is not only attenuated but is stretched as a result of the varying propagation times of different parts of the energy contained within it. As the beam is scanned across the skull this stretching of the pulse will also vary in degree. Nevertheless the consequent degradation of resolution in range is relatively insignificant in comparison with the much grosser degradation of resolution in the lateral dimension encountered by any scanning technique through the skull.

It will be appreciated that since both the incongruity of the display and the degraded resolution in range and the lateral dimensions is a consequence of the acoustic properties of the skull and especially its marked difference in acoustic impedance in comparison with soft tissue, it will be relatively difficult to overcome these problems by improvements in the engineering or electronics of the generating or receiving systems since these are not the source of the fundamental difficulties.

It will now be appreciated why, a quarter of a century after attempts were first made to image the brain with two dimensional ultrasonic pulse-echo techniques, no such images of diagnostic value have yet been achieved. Obviously investigators who have devoted much time, effort and money to the development of such scanning techniques were reluctant to acknowledge failure so that these attempts have only slowly decreased during the 1970's during which period investigators hoped that, with various modifications, they might be able to circumvent the problems.

Perhaps one of the most dramatic demonstrations that it is indeed the adult skull that prevents adequate imaging of the brain with ultrasonic reflection techniques, is the comparison between the excellent and detailed tomographs of the fetal and neonatal brain that can be obtained with ordinary B-scanning equipment (Figs. 10 & 11) in contrast to the inadequate images obtained in the adult (Figs. 2 & 3). The fetus and newborn have thin skulls which are neither ossified nor contain cancellous diploe and have an acoustic impedance very similar to that of soft tissue. Thus they offer little impediment to the imaging of the fetal and neonatal brain. However, as the child grows and its skull becomes more ossified with the formation of the cancellous diploe the situation progressively deteriorates.

Another demonstration of the obscuring effects of the skull even in children was given by Galicich et al. (1965). They studied mostly children at the Children's Hospital

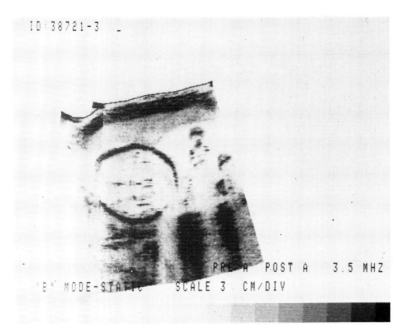

Fig. 10. Intra-uterine scan of a foetal head in horizontal section. The forehead is to the right and the median cerebral fissure and third ventricle can be seen in the median plane with the medial walls of the frontal horns of the lateral ventricles just anteriorly and to either side of the third ventricle. The twin echoes placed more laterally are the temporal horns of the lateral ventricles. This figure was made by and is reproduced by kind permission of Dr. Eric Sauerbrei.

Medical Centre, Peter Brent Brigham Hospital. Their study was a retrospective one in which the nature, size and localisation of the lesion had previously been determined prior to the ultrasonic examination which was then repeated until the investigators felt that the ultrasonic tomogram did display a lesion of appropriate size and localisation. Unfortunately they did not give the ages of the children they studied. As mentioned, in very young children, the ultrasonic examination is less unsatisfactory than in adults but deteriorates progressively as childhood advances. Nevertheless, they were only able to display subdural haematomata in two out of eight patients and cerebral metastases in none out of three. Even when a large primary supratentorial brain tumour was present, they could, with patience, only reproduce this lesion on their ultrasonic scans in eleven out of fourteen patients. Obviously, if it is so difficult with ultrasonic tomography to display retrospectively lesions which are known to exist in children where the skull imposes less of a barrier than in adults, it will be appreciated how much

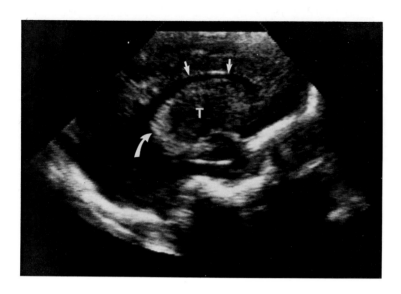

Fig. 11. Scan in the sagittal para-median plane of a neonatal brain showing the cavity of the lateral ventricle (arrows) containing the choroid plexus (curved arrow) and surrounding the thalamus (T). This scan was made by and is reproduced by kind permission of Dr. Eric Sauerbrei.

more difficult, and indeed up to the present moment impossible, it will be to display prospectively unknown lesions in adults with sufficient certainty to be of diagnostic significance.

These then are the reasons why, after a quarter of a century of endeavour, ultrasonic pulse-echo reflection techniques are not useful for the clinical diagnosis of tumours in the adult brain.

REFERENCES

Ballantine, H.T., Ludwig, G.D., Bolt, R.H. and Hueter, T. F. (1950): Ultrasonic localization of the cerebral ventricles. Trans. Amer. Neurol. Ass., 75, 38.
Galicich, J.H., Lombroso, C.T. and Matson, D.D. (1965): Ultrasonic B-scanning of the brain. J. Neurosurg., 22, 499.
Leksell, L. (1956): Echo-encephalography: Detection of intracranial complications following head injury. Acta chir. scand., 110, 301.
Moore, G. (1955): U.S. Atomic Energy Commission studies in methods in instruments to improve the localization of radioactive materials in the body with special reference to the diagnosis of brain tumours and the use of ultrasonic techniques. AECU-3012, University of Minnesota Press.

White, D.N. (1976): The Effect of the Skull upon the Spatial and Temporal Distribution of a Generated and Reflected Ultrasonic Beam. Ultramedison, Kingston, Canada.

White, D.N., Curry, G.R. and Stevenson, R.J. (1978): The acoustic characteristics of the skull. Ultrasound Med. Biol., 4, 225.

White, D.N. (1981): Pulsatile echoencephalography. Ultrasound Med. Biol., 7, 335.

# ULTRASOUND DIAGNOSIS OF THE THYROID

L. Carlier, T. Goodfellow and V.R. McCready

*Hôpital Civil de Charleroi, Belgium and The Royal Marsden Hospital, Sutton, U.K.*

Carcinoma of the thyroid is an uncommon disease, accounting for 0.7% of all cancers in females, and 0.2% in males (1). However thyroid goitres are relatively common, and the identification of a malignant goitre amidst numerous apparently benign goitres has always been a problem facing the clinician. A Leading Article (2) recommended early thyroid surgery for single thyroid nodules in females less than 40 years, and in all males based on the findings of Veith et al. (3). Although this policy has been questioned by Jackson and Thompson (4), Taylor also advised the removal of all hypo-functioning solitary thyroid nodules (5). This view was confirmed by Hoffman et al. who stated that 'there is no way of differentiating benign from malignant thyroid nodules' (6).

Many of the series reporting thyroid carcinoma originate from specialist centres. Consequently the figures do not give a true indication of the ratio of benign to malignant goitres in general clinical practice (7). However, Campbell and Sage (8) in a review of 20 years experience of thyroid cancer in a district general hospital found an overall operative incidence of 4.25% (i.e. 45 cases in 1058 thyroidectomies) with another 9 cases which did not come to surgery. In 61.1% of these cases the carcinoma presented in a form indistinguishable from that of benign goitres. It is clear, therefore, that although the figures differ from series to series, the vast majority of operations for goitre are performed for benign disease, although there may be other indications for surgery.

The advent of radioisotope scanning and ultrasonography has considerably changed the preoperative diagnosis of thyroid goitres. Scintiscanning is performed after the administration of either radioactive iodine, or Technetium 99m ($^{99}Tc^m$ pertechnetate). The appearance of the scan depends on the functional status of the tissue, and since cancerous tissue usually functions less well than normal tissue, the scan appearance is usually that of an area of reduced activity or 'cold' nodule (9).

However scintiscanning has severe limitations. It

is unable to distinguish a cold area due to a carcinoma
from one due to an adenoma, a cyst or a colloid nodule.
Resolving capacity is limited to lesions over 1 cm in
diameter and in some cases the presence of a cold nodule
may be obscured by overlying normal tissue.

The use of ultrasound scanning as a means of imaging
the thyroid is now well established (10,11,12,13). The
anatomy of the gland can be easily identified, including
its relationship to adjacent structures in the neck.
The thyroid parenchyma returns uniform echoes, with an
even echo texture. The changes that may take place in
thyroid disease are those of size, shape, regularity
of outline, and in the uniformity of the parenchymal
echoes. The echo texture may be altered (i.e. the size
and spacing of the echoes) as may be the attenuating
properties of the tissue. Displacement or invasion of
adjacent structures may also occur. However, none of
these features are specific for carcinoma, with the
exception of frank invasion of adjacent tissues.
Consequently it is difficult often to make a definitive
diagnosis of carcinoma, or indeed to exclude it.

Carlier et al. have used the technique of ultrasonic
densitometry, combined with scintigraphy, in diagnosing
thyroid swellings (14). By using a digital B-mode scanner
with 32 grey scales and a 5 MHz transducer focussed at
3 cms, images are obtained of the thyroid. By the use
of data processing, a predetermined area of tissue is
selected, and a histogram of the echo intensities within
the grey scale is constructed. The percentage of echoes
is given on the y axis and columns representing the grey
levels on the x axis. Using the histograms obtained,
they have attempted to characterise abnormal thyroid
tissue (Fig. 1).

They classified the patterns into 4 categories:-
focal (or solid) lesions, cystic lesions, multiple (or
mixed cystic and solid lesions) and diffuse lesions.
However they concluded that the technique was unable
to distinguish between benign and malignant nodules.

MATERIALS AND METHODS

A series of 870 thyroid ultrasound examinations
were performed at the Royal Marsden Hospital, Sutton,
between January 1978 and December 1980 using a linear
5MHz transducer focussed at 7.5 cms. Scanning was carried
out through a water bath. Nearly all the patients had
an isotope scan prior to the ultrasound using $^{99}Tc^m$
pertechnetate and a gamma camera with a pinhole aperture.
During this period, a total of 40 cases of carcinoma
were seen (4.6%). Histological confirmation was obtained
in each case. The isotope scans and the ultrasound scans
of these cases were reviewed, and a comparison made of
the results.

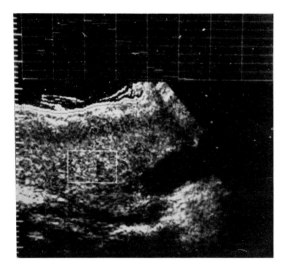

Figure 1   Simple goitre


RESULTS

A total of 27 isotope scans (67.5%) showed hypo-functioning nodules in the gland.  A further 2 cases showed hyper-functioning nodules.  The remainder (scan negative) were either normal, equivocal, showed no uptake, or were not done for various reasons.


TABLE 1. Thyroid carcinoma: isotope scan appearances.

| | | |
|---|---|---|
| Cold nodules | 27 | (67.5%) |
| Hot nodules | 2 | (5.0%) |
| Normal | 3 | (7.5%) |
| Equivocal | 2 | (5.0%) |
| No uptake | 4 | (10.0%) |
| Not done | 2 | (5.0%) |
| TOTAL | 40 | |

On ultrasound scanning, a total of 30 cases (75%) were identified as probable carcinoma, or having a high risk of malignancy.  The remaining 10 cases (25%) were classified as benign or having a low risk of malignancy (Table 2).

If the results of the two investigations are combined, a total of 3 scan negative patients also had no evidence of malignancy on the ultrasound scan.  In addition one of the hyper-functioning nodules was described as a benign adenoma.  Thus, in a total of 4 cases (10%) a diagnosis of carcinoma was not indicated by either investigation.

TABLE 2. Thyroid carcinoma: ultrasound diagnosis

| | | |
|---|---|---|
| Probable carcinoma | 19 | (47.5%) |
| Solid nodule, high risk | 9 | (22.5%) |
| Adenoma, high risk | 2 | (5.0%) |
| Adenoma, low risk | 3 | (7.5%) |
| Multinodular goitre | 2 | (5.0%) |
| Normal | 4 | (10.0%) |
| Unsatisfactory scan | 1 | (2.5%) |

DISCUSSION

Thyroid ultrasound can reliably differer⁺iate between single and multiple lesions, and between cystic and solid lesions. Combined with scintigraphy it can identify high risk nodules, and some carcinomas. However there is still an appreciable number of cases when it cannot do this, 10% in our series. This risk, though small, is still significant and at present it is difficult to disagree with the policy of early surgery for cold solitary nodules. However ultrasound is able to identify some high risk lesions which are not apparent on the isotope scan, a total of 7 in this series (34.5% of all cancers), and it therefore has a real place in the management of thyroid goitres.

TABLE 3. Ultrasonic features of thyroid malignancy

| Echo intensity | | Echo distribution | |
|---|---|---|---|
| High | 3 | Homogeneous | 14 |
| Low | 24 | Heterogeneous | 21 |
| Mixed | 9 | | |

| Edge definition | | Echo texture | |
|---|---|---|---|
| Well defined | 7 | Fine | 17 |
| Poorly defined | 25 | Coarse | 7 |
| Frank invasion | 3 | Variable | 11 |

Table 3 lists some of the features examined when assessing a thyroid nodule for possible malignancy. Figures 2-5 are all examples of various types of carcinoma, and some of the above features may be seen in each of them. A "typical" carcinoma has a low echo intensity with a heterogeneous distribution and a fine echo texture. The margins of the tumour are usually poorly defined or irregular, although frank invasion is uncommon (Figs. 2-5).

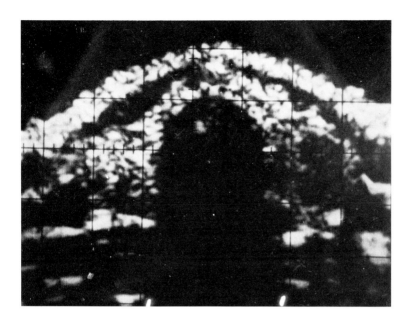

Figure 2  Medullary carcinoma

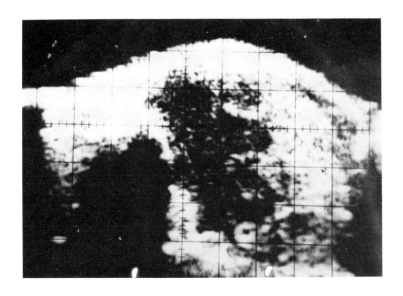

Figure 3  Anaplastic carcinoma

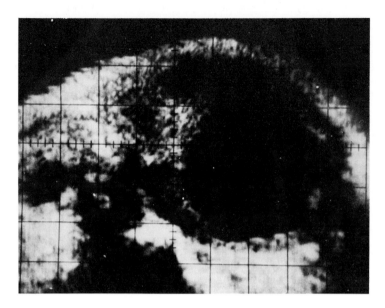

Figure 4   Follicular carcinoma

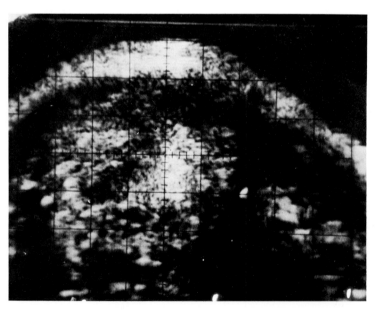

Figure 5   Papillary carcinoma

Improvement in diagnosis may be made in two directions. First, by using higher frequency transducers, e.g. 10 MHz, better resolution and recognition of malignant features may be possible, especially by studying the growing margins of the tumour. Second, by the development of tissue characterisation techniques it may be possible to obtain a more precise method of pattern recognition for normal and abnormal tissue. This could considerably improve the diagnosis, and consequently the management of the solitary thyroid nodule.

REFERENCES

1.  Waterhouse, J.A.H. (1974): In: Cancer Handbook of Epidemiology and Prognosis, p. 174. Churchill Livingstone, Edinburgh.
2.  Leading Article (1964): Br. Med. J., 2, 1022.
3.  Veith, F.J., Brooks, J.R., Grigsby, W.P. and Selenkon (1964): New Engl. J. Med., 270, 431.
4.  Jackson, I.M.D. and Thompson, J.A. (1967): Br. J. Surg. 54, 1007.
5.  Taylor, S. (1969): J. R. Coll. Surg., 14, 267.
6.  Hoffman, G.L., Thompson, N.W. and Heffron, C. (1972): Arch. Surg., 105, 379.
7.  Crile, G. and Dempsey, W.S. (1949): J.A.M.A., 139, 1247.
8.  Campbell, D.J. and Sage, R.H. (1975): Br. J. Surg., 62, 207.
9.  McCready, V.R. (1970): In: Tumours of the Thyroid Gland, p. 202. Editor: D. Smithers. Churchill Livingstone, Edinburgh.
10. Fujimoto, Y., Oka, A. and Hirose, M. (1967): Ultrasound, 5, 177.
11. Crocker, E.F., McLaughlin, A.F., Kossof, G. and Jellins, J. (1974): J. Clin. Ultrasound, 2, 305.
12. Spencer, R., Brown, M.C. and Annis, D. (1977): Br. J. Surg., 64, 841.
13. Lees, W.R., Vahl, S.P., Watson, L.R. and Russell C.G. (1978): Br. J. Surg., 65, 681.
14. Carlier, L., Becqevort, P., Dwelshauvers and Rouma, G. (1981): J. Belg. Radiol., 64, 327.

# PAROTID TUMORS AND CERVICAL ADENOPATHIES

Jean N. Bruneton[1], Maurice Sicart[2] and Francois Demard[1]

[1]*Department of Radiology and Otorhinolaryngology, Centre A. Lacas-sagne, Nice, France and* [2]*Department of Radiology, Hôpital Tripode Pellegrin, Bordeaux, France*

## I. PAROTID TUMORS

One hundred and forty one cases of parotid tumors were reviewed. In all cases, surgical and histological confirmation were obtained.

From an anatomical viewpoint, there were 110 benign tumors (73 mixed tumors, 24 cystadenolymphomas, 6 lipomas, 2 angiomas, 5 various others) and 31 malignant tumors (including 3 primary malignant lymphomas).

Two echographic criteria were employed to retain the diagnosis of a benign tumor : a tumor with a homogenic aspect and well demarcated limits. In the absence of one of these criteria, an echographic diagnosis of a malignant tumor was retained. On these bases, benign tumors (fig 1) were diagnosed correctly in 90 of the 110 cases (81.8 %) and malignant tumors (fig 2) in 21 of the 31 cases (61.8 %). The value of echography for differenciating between a benign and a malignant tumor was 79.8 %.

In addition, echography permitted correct recognition of the intra or extra-parotidean nature of an adenopathy in 62 % of 21 cases. Use for echography for investigation of parotid pathologies appears primarily warranted when faced with clinical tumefaction. Since it is at least as sensitive as sialography for such tumors, echography is sufficient to permit therapeutic decisions. Echographically-guided pucture can be carried out if a doubt subsists. In addition, utilization of high frequency transducers should improve results concerning the intra or extra-parotidean nature of adenopathies. As far as parotitis is concerned, however, when dealing with diffuse hypertrophy of the gland, echography can only confirm clinical findings and does not allow investigation of canal structure. It is in this inflammatory pathology, as well as in lithiasic conditions, that sialography retains its interest.

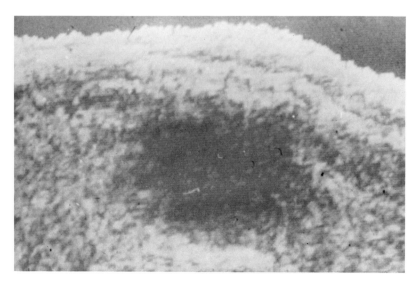

Figure 1. Mixed tumor of the parotid gland.

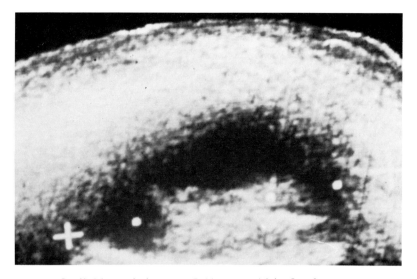

Figure 2. Malignant tumor of the parotid gland.

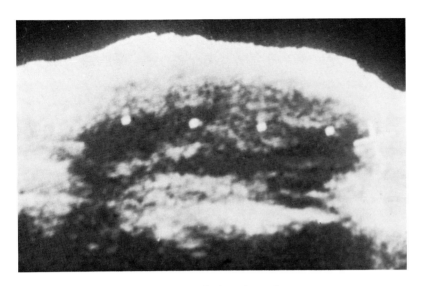

Figure 3. Metastatic cervical lymph node.

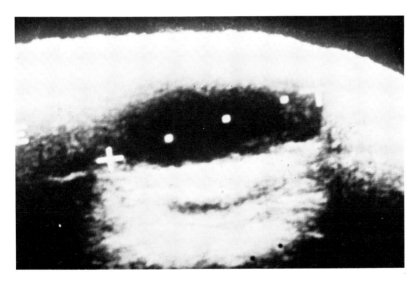

Figure 4. Non Hodgkinian lymphoma.

## II. CERVICAL ADENOPATHIES

Malignant cervical lymph node pathologies were reviewed in connection with 120 cases (100 metastatic nodes associated with an ENT cancer (fig 3) and 20 cases of malignant lymphoma (fig 4) ).

In addition to anatomical verification of all cases, each node was investigated as to its echostructure, diameter and vascular relationships, especially with the internal jugular vein.

Cervical adenopathies can be diagnosed by clinical examination, and the superficial nature of such enlarged nodes allows puncture which can orient diagnosis. Echography thus offers specific advantages in such cases.

While there is a definite difference in echostructure between lymphomatous nodes, which are almost fluid-like, and solid metastatic nodes, the interest of echography lies elsewhere. It is extremely helpful to know the exact diameter of an adenopathy in order to assess its evolution under treatment, either by chemotherapy or radiotherapy (radiotherapy almost always causes cutaneous thickening which renders clinical examination difficult). Furthermore, it is also useful to know the relationship of a voluminous adenopathy with the internal jugular and primary carotid vessels in connection with latero-cervical localizations. Indeed, it is easy to detect compression of the internal jugular vein which may or may not require angiography to decide on the surgical tactic. It is much less frequent for the primary carotid artery to be compressed or invaded by the nodal neoplastic process.

## CONCLUSION

Parotid tumors should be investigated by echography since the sensitivity of this examination allows differentiation between benign and malignant tumors ; the necessity or not of surgery can thus be evaluated. The primary role of echography when dealing with cervical adenopathies lies in the search for vascular complications, in particular concerning the internal jugular vein for voluminous nodes, and measurement of node volume allowing evaluation of response to radiotherapy or chemotherapy.

# SCREENING OF UPPER ABDOMINAL ORGANS BY DIGITAL LINEAR ARRAY REALTIME SCANNER

T. Wagai and S.E. Park

*Medical Ultrasonics Research Center, Juntendo University School of Medicine, Hongo, Bunkyo-ku, Tokyo, Japan*

The echographic realtime imaging techniques have been widely utilized with its high clinical evaluation together with remarkable technological improvement not only in the field of Cardiology and Obstetrics but also of abdominal organs as " Abdominal echography ". In Japan, particularly linear array realtime scanner has been developed rapidly and digitalization of realtime images and its TV mode display have become the standardization of equipments. In this paper, clinical application of digital linear array realtime scanner in the field of abdominal organs, particularly of the liver, gallbladder and pancreas and the satisfactory result of its screening use in this field performed at the Health Check Center are reported.

EQUIPMENT FOR LINEAR ARRAY REALTIME SCANNER

Fig.1 is the linear array realtime scanner ( SSD-250, Aloca Co.) which was applied at this series of examination. As the performance of the equipment, length of the probe is 10cm, number of multi-element are 400 and frequency is 3.5MHz. Digital display of realtime images with 512X512 matrix, grey scale performance by 5 bit, standard TV mode display with 384 or 256 scanning line according to magnification function and 4 steps electric dynamic focusing system are applied. Resolution is under 2mm in both axial and lateral direction and scanning speed is 30 frams per second. According to these performances, improvement of realtime images, easy freezing of images, simultaneous display of two continued or differently directed images and directional electric recording of VTR are available and these advantages are useful and effective for clinical application, particularly for the screening use.

For the abdominal echography, manual contact scanning technique has been usually applied and recently, automatic mechanical compound scanner with water path technique has been widely applied. Furthermore, various improvements have been achieved even in these equipments such as digitalization of images and combination of realtime scanner with manual contact scanning technique. On the other hand, linear or convex array realtime scanner has been applied rapidly with improvement of image quality, compact design,

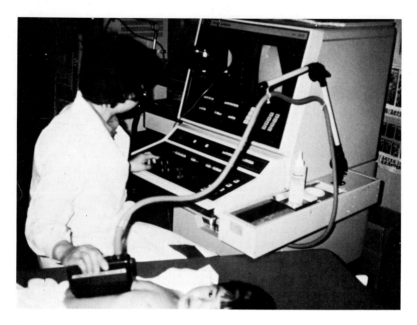

Fig.1  Linear array realtime scanner ( SSD -250, Aloca Co. )

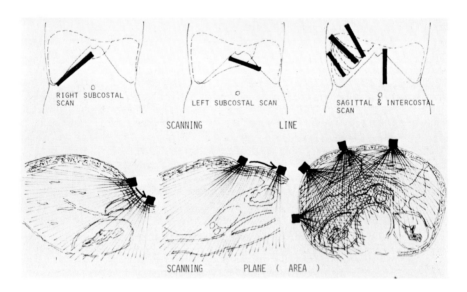

Fig.2 Position of scanner and echographic planes for screening
of upper abdominal organs

easy procedure, particularly for the abdominal echography.

ECHOGRAPHIC IMAGES OF UPPER ABDOMINAL ORGANS

Position and direction of echographic plane are selected for abdominal echography as shown in Fig.2 according
to organs examined. As the width of images is not enough
to cover whole area of upper abdominal organs, scanner has
to be moved continuously changing its position, direction
and angle as shown in this figure. Several examples of
echographic images of the gallbladder, liver and pancreas
by linear array realtime scanner are demonstrated.
Fig.3 is two cases of cholelithiasis obtained by
right intercostal approach. The easy freezing function of
realtime images was effective for the examination of the
gallbladder. Dignostic accuracy of cholelithiasis was more
than 90% and it was superior than X-ray cholecystography.
At the same time, echographic detection of gallstones has
been considered the most suitable indication at the screening in this field with various clinical advantages. Fig.4
is two cases of gallbladder carcinoma. The gallbladder
carcinoma was detected by the images of irregularily thickened wall and or abnormal tissue images prominenced from
the wall which was different from stone images. As the
majority of gallbladder carcinoma cases combined with
gallstone, in cholelithiasis, these findings have to be
carefully examined. The gallbladder polyp was also detected
very often. Concerning the common bile duct, imaging in
normal case was possible but difficult generally compared
with the gallbladder. In the case with dilatation, echographic imaging was more easy and stone or carcinoma in
the common bile duct were detected. Fig.5 is two cases of
common bile carcinoma. Dilatation of the common bile duct
and complete cbstruction by carcinoma tissue were clearly
demonstrated. For the echographic examination of the liver,
continued observation of the whole area by changing the

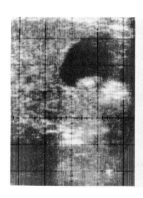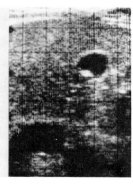

Fig.3 Echographic images
of cholelithiasis by linear
array realtime scanner,
3.5MHz

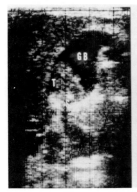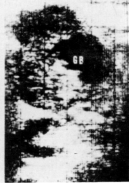

Fig.4 Echographic images of gallbladder cancer

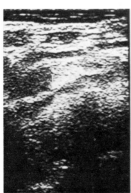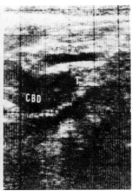

Fig.5 Echographic images of common bile duct carcinoma

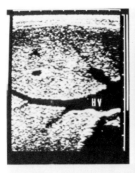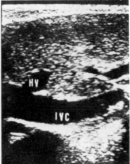

Fig.6 Echographic images of dilatation of hepatic vein and inferior vena cava

echographic plane was very important as shown in Fig.2. As
one of the advantages of the realtime scanner, easy and
clear imaging of various vessels was indicated. In the
liver, the hepatic vein, portal vein and the inferior vena
cava were easily detected and analysis of these vessels
were effective for the diagnosis of diffuse and space occupying lesions. Fig.6 is two cases of dilatation of the
hepatic vein and inferior vena cava by the disturbance of
venous return. Fig.7 is two cases of dilatation of the
intrahepatic bile ducts and easy detection of such finding
was very useful for the differential diagnosis of extra-
hepatic obstructive jaundice and for the echo-guided puncture. Fig.8 is two cases of liver cirrhosis. Fine irregular
margin of the liver, thin and irregularily waved hepatic
vein and image of ascites were characteristic in liver
cirrhosis. High level of intrahepatic echo, change of the
hepatic vein and increased ultrasonic attenuation were
useful for detecting liver cirrhosis at early stage.

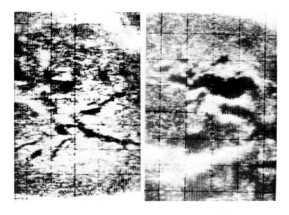

Fig.7 Echographic images
of dilatation of intra-
hepatic bile duct

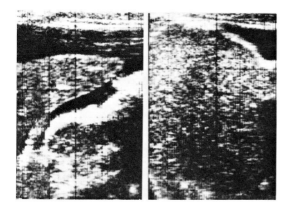

Fig.8 Echographic images
of liver cirrhosis

83

Detection of space occupying lesions in the liver was the
most expectable indication of the echography. Fig.9 is
two cases of liver cyst. As cystic disease in the liver
showes no clinical symptom in its early stage, echography
was very important in the series of echographic screening
for the detection of these cystic disease. At the same
time, echography was effective for the differential diagnosis of congenital jaundice in baby, particularly for the
detection of congenital common bile duct dilatation(cyst).
The early detection of liver cancer has been important
subject. Fig.10 is two cases of small early metastatic
liver cancer with approximately 2cm in diameter. Solid
mass images with high echo level and irregular margin and
loop configulation of the hepatic vein arround tumors by
the pressure of tumors were characteristic in the metastatic liver cancer. Primary liver cancer, hepatoma ( Fig.11)
showed more complicated images such as mass images with
low echo level, irregular internal echo content with halo
image and intratumor vascularization. Early detection of

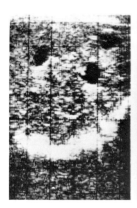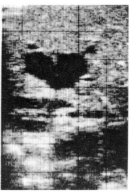

Fig.9 Echographic images
of liver cyst

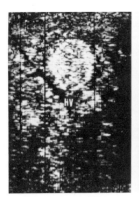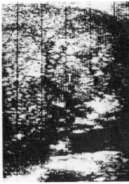

Fig.10 Echographic images
of early metastatic liver
cancer

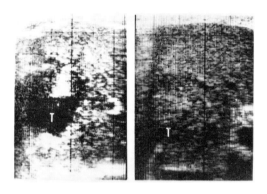

Fig.11 Echographic images
of primary liver cancer
( hepatoma )

pancreas cancer is the most important and difficult subject
in the field of gastroenterology. Concerning the imaging
of the pancreas, detection of various vessels around the
pancreas is necessary. The linear array realtime scanner
was effective for such purpose compared with other echographic imaging technique. Fig.12 is two cases of chronic
pancreatitis. Swelling of the pancreas with smooth margin
and homogeneous internal echo content were characteristic.
Fig.13 is two cases of early pancreas head cancer. Localized swelling of the pancreas head with irregular margin
and with homogeneous or localized irregular internal echo
content and interruption of the pancreatic duct were characteristic in the pancreas cancer.

ECHOGRAPHIC SCREENING OF UPPER ABDOMEN

    According to these superior clinical results, echo-
graphic realtime imaging technique has been considered a
suitable screening tool for upper abdominal organs such as

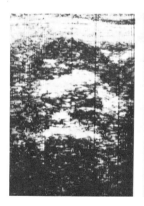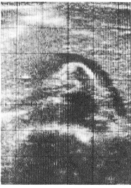

Fig.12 Echographic images
of chronic pancreatitis

85

the liver, gallbladder, pancreas, kidney, spleen, abdominal
aorta and others. Such project has been carried out since
1977 for the early detection of diseases in these organs,
particularly cancer at the Health Check Center ( Doyukai
Clinik, Tokyo ). At the Center, as various functional and
morphological examinations are performed in a short period
of one or one and half days, echographic examination also
had to be carried out rapidly during these busy scheduled
programs. After various trials, I have applied linear
array realtime scanner as shown in Fig.14. The echographic
examination has been performed in the morning without taking breakfast at sitting position. In practice, echographic
examination was performed immediately after drinking sugar
solution which was 150ml for blood sugar tolerance test.
Such position and drinking sugar solution was effective
for obtaining clear images of abdominal organs, particularly of the pancreas through the antrum of stomach in
spite of such small amount of solution. Procedure of echographic examination was carried out by sonographers under
the fixed manual as shown in Fig.15.

In the procedure (1), scanner was placed firstly at
the middle part of the left costal arch and echographic
plane was directed toward the diaphragm and then, echographic plane was continuously changed by sector and parallel movement of scanner along the illustrated line until
the middle abdomen. During the scanning procedure (1),
transverse images of left lobe of the liver, splenic vein,
portal vein, abdominal aorta, inferior vena cava and the
pancreas were recorded by VTR. After that, procedure (2)
and (3) were performed with similar technique and through
these procedure, right lobe of the liver, hepatic vein,
portal vein in the liver, gallbladder and the right kidney
were recorded. Procedure (4) was longitudinal imaging of
the upper abdomen. Furthermore, in the case with insufficient imaging of the liver and gallbladder, right intercostal scanning procedure was added. These recording of
continued realtime images by VTR were performed within

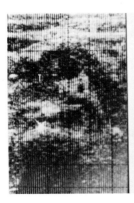 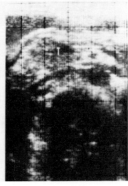

Fig.13 Echographic images
of early pancreas head
cancer

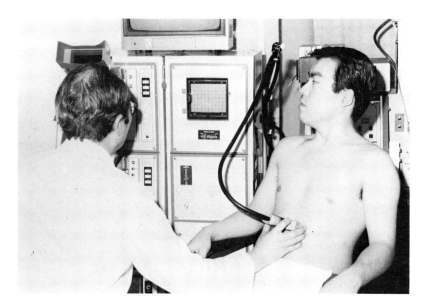

Fig.14   Screening of upper abdominal organs by linear array
         realtime scanner

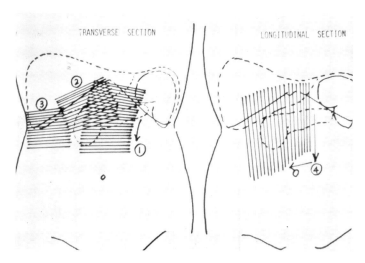

Fig.15   Procedure of echographic screening of upper abdominal
         organs

three minute and echographic screening of upper abdomen
for one applicant was completed within 4 or 5 minutes.

RESULT OF ECHOGRAPHIC SCREENING OF UPPER ABDOMEN

As the Health Check Center is for checking health
condition of adults, approximately 70% of applicants were
50 to 60 years old generation who were almost healthy and
without any soecial symptoms. Table 1 is the result of
echographic screening of upper abdomen on 8298 cases by
applying the technique stated before during the last two
years. These results were confirmed by following precise
examination technique such as X-ray CT, angiography, biopsy and others. The most high incidence was cholelithiasis
which was 244 cases ( approximately 3% ). In 70 years old
generation, it was about 10%. Detecting accuracy of cholelithiasis by echography was superior than X-ray cholecystography which was performed at the same time. The result
was important and interesting clinically, because almost
all cases were so called the silent stone which showed no
clinical symptom before. It was also interesting that
cystic disease in the kidney and liver were detected at
relatively high rate with 0.78 and 0.55% respectively. As
these cases showed no clinical symptoms and no abnormal
laboratory datas, echographic screening was effective for
detecting such morphological changes. Furthermore, 4 cases
of liver cancer, two cases of liver cirrhosis, one case of
aneurysm of the abdominal aorta, one case of pancreatic

RESULT OF ECHOGRAPHIC SCREENING OF UPPER ABDOMEN
- 8298 cases -

| | | | |
|---|---|---|---|
| CHOLELITHIASIS | 244(2.94%) | HIGH LEVEL INTRAHEPATIC ECHO | 114 |
| KIDNEY CYST | 65(0.78%) | DILATATION OF HEPATIC VEIN | 55 |
| LIVER CYST | 46(0.55%) | ABNORMAL SHAPE OF PANCREAS | 39 |
| HEPATOMEGALY | 17 | DILATATION OF IVC | 20 |
| SPLENOMEGALY | 6 | ENLARGEMENT OF GALLBLADDER | 15 |
| LIVER CANCER | 4 | TOTAL | 243 |
| LIVER CIRRHOSIS | 2 | | |
| ANEURYSM OF ABDOMINAL AORTA | 2 | | |
| PANCREATIC CYST | 1 | | |
| GALLBLADDER CANCER | 1 | | |
| ADRENAL GLAND TUMOR | 1 | | |
| TOTAL | 389 | NO. WITH ABNORMAL FINDINGS | 632 |
| | | | ( 7.6% ) |

cyst, one case of gallbladder cancer and others were detected. In addition to these findings, high level of intrahepatic echo which was closely related to fatty liver, liver cirrhosis and diffuse chronic liver disease, abnormal shape and swelling of the pancreas and others were detected. However, as these morphological findings were firstly experienced by echographic screening, these cases have been followed by repeated echographic examinations and by other diagnostic techniques.

In recent years, various body imaging modalities such as X-ray CT, RCT, NMR, digital radiography and others have shown excellent clinical results for detecting cancer with rapid technological improvement. However, these new modalities are not always suitable for the screening of cancer because of their examination procedure and econocal point of view. Echographic examination will be expected for the screening of cancer even in future based on the results obtained in this series. Under such situations, echographic equipments, particularly designed for the screening use with automation function and other superior performances are extremely expected.

REFERENCES

1. Wagai,T. and Kobayashi,M. (1979 ) : Diagnostic criteria of ultrasonic pancreatic cancer images and its clinical evaluation, p.94, Report of 2nd WFUMB meeting, Miyazaki
2. Sakuma,K., Wagai,T. et al ( 1979 ) : Screening of liver, gallbladder and pancreas diseases by ultrasonic real-time imaging technique in the Health Check Center, p. 106, Report of 2nd WFUMB meeting, Miyazaki
3. Wagai,T. and Park, S.E. et al ( 1979 ) : Investigation of ultrasonic image of hepatic vein for the diagnosis of diffuse liver diseases, p. 270, Report of 2nd WFUMB meeting, Miyazaki
4. Wagai, T. and Park, S. E. ( 1980 ) : Digital linear array realtime scanner and its screening use of abdominal organ diseases, p. 21, 10th Annual meeting of Australian Society for Ultrasound in Medicine, Sydney

# ULTRASOUND IN THE DIAGNOSIS AND MANAGEMENT OF PANCREATIC CANCER

F.S. Weill and P. Rohmer

*Department of visceral Radiology, University Hospital (C.H.U.), Besancon 25000, France*

## 1 - DIAGNOSIS :

### 1-1 : Examination technique :

The classical sonographic examination technique is based on manual B-scanning of the supine patient. However, since in the supine position air in the bowel often constitutes an obstacle to the progression of the ultrasonic beam, classical B-scanning is unable to display the body and tail of the pancreas in at least 30% of patients. This is why Kossof (1978) has proposed automatic scanning in the prone position, after gastric filling with methyl-cellulose.

We use the real-time technique, with a mechanical real-time head. This permits scanning on the recumbent patient, but also in the erect position, in which intestinal gas moves up to the colonic flexures. With this technique, using also gastric filling (and, whenever necessary, complementary positionings, as left lateral decubitus) the entire pancreas can be displayed even in fat patients. Our rate of failure, even regarding the pancreatic tail, is only 1%. (19).

We advise examining the fasting patient : when filling is necessary, we give the patient mashed vegetables soup (Eisencher, 1980) rather than methyl-cellulose, since it is better accepted.

The procedure begins with sagittal parallel sections of the epigastrium. Sweeping transverse scans are then carried out, from the xyphoïd process, down and back up. Real-time permits one to correct the scanning plane if the first scans show the pancreas to have an oblique orientation. Right intercostal sections display the gallbladder, common bile duct, and liver.

Left coronal and intercostal sections show the caudal region, the spleen and left kidney. The pancreatic tail can also be studied by posterior transrenal scanning, readily performed on the standing patient after the epigastric cuts.

Of course, pancreatic scanning represents part of a comprehensive sonological-clinical examination. This means that the entire biliary tree and liver (dilatation, deposits) are also examined, as well as the neighbouring retroperitoneal compartments (evaluation of the tumoral extension, assessment of the mesenteric, vessels screening for adenopathies) and splenic vessels, and of the I.V.C. Far from being a time consuming procedure, such a comprehensive

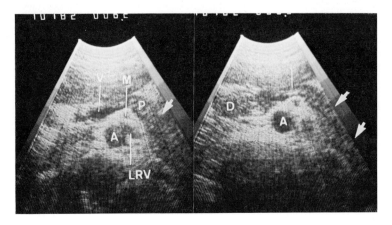

FIG 1 : Normal pancreas. Two parallel real-time transverse
sections in erect position.
     A – The pancreas (P) is surrounded by more echogenic
fat. Note good delineation of body and tail (arrow), and vascular relationships :
          V : splenoportal confluence ; M : S M A
          A : aorta ; L R V : left renal vein.
    Iso reflective prepancreatic area  is hepatic.

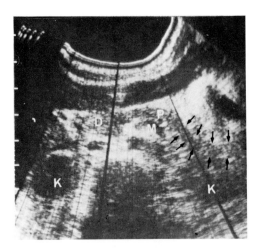

FIG 2 :         Normal pancreas. (P) – transverse manual
                      scanning.
     Pancreas, surrounded by fat is displayed posterior to
liver. White spot within hepatic parenchyma corresponds to fal-
ciform ligament. Note again delineation of body and tail
(arrows). Pseudomass close to pancreatic head corresponds to
descending part of duodenum. (D) (M : S M A ; K : kidneys).
(Courtesy, Mosby publ. ST Louis, U.S.A.).

examination, requires only, if one uses a good real-time machine, for five minutes.

We use classical B-scanning only as a complementary procedure, in case of large pancreatic masses in fact rather to obtain documents more similar to CT scans, than to help the diagnostic procedure itself.

1-2 : The normal pancreas :

The normal pancreas is displayed in front of the large vessels as a sausage-shaped reflective element, notched at the level of its neck by the adjacent mesenteric vessels. The portal vein give rise to a deep groove in the posterior aspect of the gland (fig 1). The shape of the pancreas is harmonious. Its contours are smooth, but can be marked by a light scalloping which is also demonstrated by CT scanning. The uncinate process is visualized posterior to the S M V.

The pancreas is surrounded by fat, which is usually markedly more reflective than the pancreatic tissue. Conversely, on CT scans, fat is much more transparent than the pancreas : hence the outstanding contrast of pancreatic contours on CT scans, compared to sonographic patterns. With some training however, the fatty boundaries of the gland are quite clearly appreciated on sonograms. (fig 1 and 2). Regarding the pancreatic tissue itself, ultrasound gives more detailed information than CT. The pancreatic tissue is homogenous and echogenic. Its reflectivity is at least equal to that of the liver, and often superior to it. The pancreatic duct is quite constantly visualized, at least as a thin reflective line.

The different relations of the pancreas, of which the list follows, are readily displayed :
- Stomach and duodenum (fig 2 and 3 A).
- Common bile duct
- Vascular elements :
  ° aorta and vena cava
  ° celiac trunk and its division in hepatic
and splenic artery.
  ° splenic vein, splenoportal junction and
portal vein.
  ° superior mesenteric vein and artery
  ° left renal vein and artery.

The proximal relationship existing between the body and tail of the pancreas on the one hand, and the left renal vessels on the other hand must be emphasized : they demonstrate the transverse pancreatic orientation existing in 60% of subjects (Weill, 1980).

1-3 : Pancreatic tumors : carcinomas

_Indirect signs :
  ° In tumors of the pancreatic head, an early sign is

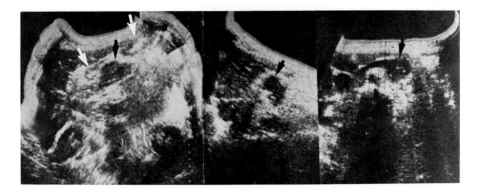

FIG 3 : Pancreatic carcinomas.
    A B - First patient.
    A - transverse section shows sonolucent mass with
pseudopod-like extensions (black arrow). Note echogenicity of
peri-pancreatic fat. Note also typical bull'eye pattern of
adjacent stomach. (white arrows)
    B - sagittal section shows mass anterior to aorta. (A).
    C - transverse section in another patient shows mass
in pancreatic body (arrow) (G : gall bladder).

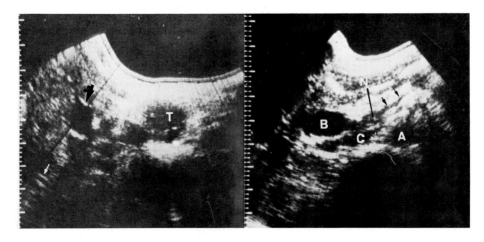

FIG 4 : Pancreatic carcinoma. Binoma sign.
    A - transverse scan shows tumor (T). Note dilated in-
fundibulum of gallbladder (black arrow) and dilated intrahepatic ducts. (white arrow).
    B - Parallel more cranial scan shows on each side of
tumoral nodule (N) dilated common bile duct (B) and dilated
pancreatic duct (arrows). ( C vena cava, A : aorta).

often the dilatation of the common bile duct. Dilatation on
the pancreatic duct is also encountered. Associated dilatation of
both ducts constitutes a relevant sign of juxtapapillary tumor.
("binoma sign") (fig 4 ) (18).

We consider the common bile duct as dilated if larger
than half the diameter of the neighbouring portal vein. (13).
The pancreatic duct should not bewider than 4 mm.
° the I.V.C. ans S M V are flattened.

Direct ultrasonic signs of carcinomas :
Following  are the main sonographic features of pancreatic tumors :
- a mass, bulging outside  of the normal parenchymal
boundaries.
- smooth contours, with, in 50% of cases, small pseu-
dopod like extensions.
- in 96% of cases a sonolucent echotexture, with a few
scattered echoes, or a few large reflective foci. (fig 3 to 5). In
4% of cases only the tumoral echotexture is strongly reflective (12).

The delineation between the tumoral tissue and the
adjacent normal pancreatic tissue if usually well marked. Since,
as mentioned above, the usual echotexture of carcinomas is poorly
echogenic, pseudopod-like extension are well outlined against the
reflective peripancreatic fat.

In case of jaundice, proper scans display the pattern
of the choledocal stop

A particular pattern appears when the tumoral process
arises from the uncinate process:such a tumor developes posteriorly
to the S M V, and pushes the vessel forward along with the
normal pancreas, as would do a lymphomatous lymphnode for instance.

Adenopathies :
Metastatic adenopathies can be displayed adjacent to
the pancreas of infiltrating the hepatoduodenal ligament, in the
vicinity of the portal vein and common bile duct, or close to
the celiac trunk.

1 - 4 : Other kind of tumors :
Cystadenomas (Weill, 1973, Wolson, 1976) have different
patterns according to their contents in cystic elements and to the
cysts'size : cystadenomas with large cysts can look like pseudocysts if no intracystic growth is demonstrated. Cystadenomas with
multiple smaller cysts have a rather typical multilocular appearance. Cystadenomas in which solid  areas are predominant have a
unspecific pattern.
Secreting apudomas are usually to small to be visualized
on sonoscans. The size of non-secreting apudoma is greater. They
appear as rounded, well limited, more or less echogenic masses.

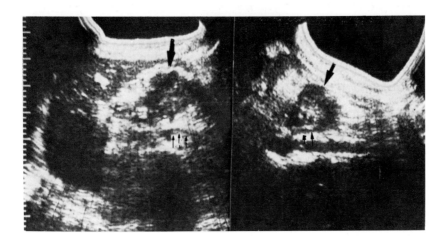

FIG 5 : Pancreatic carcinoma. Study of extension.
           A - Transverse scan : fat separates tumor (broad arrow)
from left renal vein. (small arrow).
           B - Sagittal scan . S M A (arrowhead) is close to mass.


1 - 5 Pitfalls and limitation of ultrasonic diagnosis :

        A gross pitfall arises from pseudomasses of digestive
origin. To avoid confusion it is commendable to check such masses by
follow-up examinations, or by an prolonged real-time examination.
Such pseudomasses change in shape and size. A "brownian movement"
due to gas bubbles  or digestive elements can be observed inside
the mass. (Weill, 1979). This sign is enhanced by fluid ingestion.

        Limitations intrinsic to the ultrasonic diagnosis itself
constitute a much graver set-back : ultrasonic  images are macroscopic and not histologic.

        We have seen above that the appearance of some cystade-
nomas is similar to that of pseudocysts. Similarly, inflammatory
nodules can mimick tumoral nodules : inflammatory nodules can also
be sonolucent ; they can also be  acompanied by a dilatation of
the pancreatic duct (however, in 60% of inflammatory dilatations,
the pancreatic duct has a particular "zipper-like" pattern (16) ;
lastly the clinical history accompanying such nodules can be
exactly that of a carcinoma,with loss of weight, pain and also
jaundice or haemorrage due to splenic vein thrombosis.

        Retroperitoneal lymphnodes push the S M V and splenic
vein forward, whereas pancreatic masses bring about posterior venous
compression. But, as we saw above, tumors originating from the
uncinate process behave as do lymphnodes.

        All those limitations explain why pancreatic puncture,
developed by H.H. Holm, S. Hancke and Rasmussen (3, 4, 5) has
become so widely utilized.

1 - 6 : Pancreatic puncture :
         Technique : a fine puncture needle is guided  into
the pancreatic mass by the mean of an ultrasonic device after local
anesthesia. There are two kinds of guiding devices :
                    - one is   a tunnelized classical B-scan transducer
                    - the other is based on real-time :
                              ° some adapt a lateral guiding device on a
sector scanner,
                              ° in others, the needle is inserted in a
tunnelized linear array.

         According to H.H. Holm and Hancke, accidents and inci-
dents are extremely rare. A fatal pancreatitis has however been
reported by Evans and associates (1981). Provided a good cytologic
diagnosis is available, puncture permits one to reach a precise
diagnosis in a matter of hours after a primary ultrasonic diagnosis
of pancreatic mass has been achieved.  Guided puncture also permits
pancreatography by injection of contrast medium  in the pancreatic
duct (1) . Ultrasonic guidance can also facilitate percutaneous
cholangiography.

   2 - RESULTS :   DIAGNOSTIC VALUE  OF  ULTRASOUND  IN PANCREATIC
MASSES - SCREENING.
         In a series of 83 patients, TAYLOR and assoc. (1981)
report a sensivity of 94% and a specificity of 99%. In a personal
series of 266 patients, we had a succes rate of 94% in the diagnosis
of pancreatic masses. However these results concern only large masses.
We know of no statistical study concerning small masses only (under
4 cm), or caudal masses only. Gastric filling and intercostal scanning   should however permit equivalent results regarding this particular tumoral location. Similar results have been published by
Lackner and assoc. (1981), who compared ultrasound and CT : both
methods achieved similar results, except in chronic pancreatitis,
where CT better visualized tiny calcified foci.

         Wagaï (1978) has proposed mass screening of pancreatic
carcinoma by the means of an ultrasound equiped ambulance. Such
a facility is easy to obtain since most real-time machines are
portable  or at least mobile. We have personnaly scanned over
15 000 patients. We have found in asymptomatic patients many
liver tumors, renal carcinomas, retroperitoneal lymphnodes, and
even  digestive carcinomas - but only one pancreatic carcinoma.
So finally, true screening in asymptomatic patients seems rather
disappointing. But the reliability of ultrasound in the diagnosis
of pancreatic masses is not questionable. Guided puncture is however
necessary to achieve a specific diagnosis.

   3 - STAGING   OF  PANCREATIC  CARCINOMA - RELATIONS OF ULTRA-
SOUND  CT AND OTHER  PROCEDURES :

   3 - 1 : Local and regional extension  - CT :
         We already underscored the particular contrast existing
in CT between the peripancreatic fat and the pancreatic parenchyma.

Generally speaking, CT displays better than ultrasound
the organ  contours. Thus CT is superior to ultrasound in the evaluation of a local  or regional tumoral extension, as for instance  -
involvement of the gastric wall or splenic parenchyma.

However a thorough analysis, of the peripancreatic
fact and adjacent vessels.permits also ultrasonic evaluation of the
tumoral extension. (fig 5 ). Regarding the visualization of small
intraparenchymal nodules,  ultrasound achieves better results
than  CT. It is therefore possible to advocate ultrasound for
primary diagnosis, reserving to CT two kinds of indications:

- primary diagnosis after an insufficient or ambiguous
sonography.
- complementary studies regarding tumoral extension,
once ultrasound has shown a mass and guided puncture confirmed
malignancy.

3 - 2 : P.T.C. - - E.R.C.P. :

Is it necessary to carry out    P.T.C.    in all cases of
jaundice due to pancreatic carcinoma ? Certainly not in our opinion.
P T C is useful in case of diagnostic discrepancy, or when ultrasound has shown a hilar obstruction. In jaundice due to cephalic
carcinoma, the ultrasonic pattern of ductal dilatation is so typical
that in most cases (92% in a series of 199 jaundices- Weill, 1979),
the positive diagnosis of dilatation the diagnosis of leve. of obstruction and the diagnosis of cause of obstruction are readily
achieved.
Neither retrograde cholangiography nor wirsungography have
indications in the field of pancreatic masses. E  R C P can however
be used as a complementary diagnostic procedure in patients whose
history is consistant with pancreatic carcinoma, whereas ultrasound
and CT were negative.

3 - 3 Liver metastases :   Ultrasonic liver scanning constitutes the best procedure in order to screen for liver metastases.

3 - 4 : Follow-up : ultrasound if perfectly suited to
monitor the tumoral evolution by follow up examinations. Ultrasonic
monitoring  is however less rewarding in pancreatic carcinoma than
in other tumors, due to the poor prognosis of this particular
neoplasm.

4 - ULTRASOUND IN THE MANAGEMENT OF PANCREATIC CARCINOMA :
Ultrasound could be used in the field of radiotherapic
dosimetry. CT is however more precise with that regard since it
better displays tumoral contours. In fact, since radiotherapy is
poorly efficacious in    pancreatic carcinoma, dosimetry is not a
frequent request in that particular oncologic field.

The morphological and cytological diagnosis achieved
by the mean of sonography (and complementary CT) should lead to
conservative management policies whenever the tumor is non resec-
table (large size, lymphnodes, involvement of neighbouring organs)
or even whenever, according to its size, the prognosis is poor.

Palliative surgery is justified in case of jaundice. Internal biliary derivation can be attempted in some cases. Cost,risk and disconfort definitely forbid ineffective surgery in advanced body and tail cancer.

Ultrasound is still useful in such patients in case of intense chronic pain in order to guide, as advocated by Holm ( 6 ) a needle to the sympathic ganglia, and carry out an alcoolization. Guided alcoolization is a simple and efficient antialgic procedure.

CONCLUSION :
1) Carried out with a correct technique (real-time, standing position, gastric filling if necessary), ultrasound is perfectly instrumental to show pancreatic masses.

3) Guided puncture and cytology are necessary to confirm malignancy.
4) Complementary CT is useful for staging.
5) Ultrasound is the best procedure to screen for liver deposits.
6) Once ultrasound and puncture have demonstrated a pancreatic cancer ; once ultrasound and CT have shown its non resectability, surgery must not be considered except in case of jaundice.
7) Guided puncture permits eventually antialgic alcoolization of celiac ganglia.

REFERENCES :

1 - COOPERBERG P.L., COHEN M.M., and GRAHAM M. : Ultrasonographically guided percutaneous pancreatography. Report of two cases. A.J.R. 132 : 662-663, 1979.

2 - EISENCHER A. : Personal communication (1980)

3 - EVANS W.K., CHIA-SING-HO, MC LOUGHLIN and LIANG-CHE TAO : Fatal necrotizing pancreatitis following fine needle aspiration biopsy of the pancreas. RADIOLOGY, 141, 61-62, 1981.

4 - HANCKE S., HOLM H.H., and KOCH F. : Ultrasonically guided fine needle biopsy of the pancreas. SURG. GYNECOL. OBST., 140 : 361-364, 1975.

5 - HANCKE S. : Ultrasound in the diagnosis of pancreatic cancerscanning and percutaneous fine needle biopsy. ALMQUIST and WIKSELL publ. STOCKLHOLM, 1980.

6 - HOLM H.H. and KRISTENSEN K. : Ultrasonically guided puncture technique. MUSKGAARD Publ. COPENHAGEN 1980.

7 - KOSSOF G., WARREN P., and GARRET W. : The examination of upper abdomen through the liquid filled stomach. 3nd Europ Congress of Ultrasonics in Medicine. BOLOGNA 1978, Abstracts 17-18.

8 - LACKNER K., FROMMHOLD H., GRAUNHOFF H., MODDER LL., HENSER L., BRAUN G., BAUMAN R., and SCHERER K. : Wertigkeit der computer tomographie und der sonographie innerhalb der Pankreas diagnostik. ROFO 132 : 509-513, 1980.

9 - TAYLOR K.J.W., BUCHIN P.J., VISCOMI G.N., and ROSENFIELD A.T., Ultrasonographic scanning of the pancreas. RADIOLOGY 138 : 211-213, 1981.

10 - WAGAI : Personal communication (1980).

11 - WEILL F., BECKER J.C., KRAEHENBUHL J.R., HERIOT G. et WALTER J.P. : Atlas clinique de radiographie ultrasonore. MASSON ed. PARIS 1973.

12 - WEILL F., MARMIER A., PARONNEAU P., ZELTNER F., et BOUGOINS A. : et BOURGOIN A. : Fiabilité de l'exploration ultrasonore du pancréas. Résultats de 266 observations contrôlées. JOURNAL RADIOL. 60, 9-11, 1979.

13 - WEILL F. MARMIER A., PARONNEAU P., ZELTNER F., et ROHMER P. : Etude ultrasonore des ictères. Sémiologie. Résultats à propos de 199 cas. J. RADIOL. ELECTROL. 59 : 659-688, 1979.

14 - WEILL F., ZELTNER F. ROHMER P., BIHR E., et TUETEY J.B. : Les images gastriques et intestinales en ultrasonographie abdominale. Le signe du mouvement Brownien. J. RADIOL. ELECTROL. 60 : 579-590, 1979.

15 - WEILL F., ROUX J., BARTOLI J. : Etude topographique des rapports vasculaires ultrasonores du pancréas.
         I veine splénique, artère médentérique supérieure. Veine mésentérique supérieure, tronc coeliaque. J. RADIOL. 61 : 79-87, 1980.

16 - WEILL F., BRUN Ph. et BARTOLI J. : Etude topographique des rapports vasculaires ultrasonores du pancréas.
         II artères et veines rénales. J. RADIOL. 61 85-87  1980.

17 - WEILL F. : Ultrasonography of digestive diseases. MOSBY PUBL. ST LOUIS (U.S.A.) 2nd edition 1982, (chapt 18 to 26).

18 - WEILL F., BIHR E., ZELTNER F., ROHMER P., PARONNEAU P., LO RUSSO G. : Etude ultrasonore des dilatations du canal de Wirsung. J. RADIOL. 61, 155-160, 1980.


19 - WOLSON A.H. and WALLS W.J. : Ultrasonic characteristics of cystadenoma of the pancreas. RADIOLOGY 119 : 203-205, 1976.

# ULTRASONIC DEMONSTRATION OF GASTRIC CANCER AND ITS LYMPH NODE METASTASES

Yasutsugu Bandai, Masatoshi Makuuchi, Goro Watanabe, Toru Itoh, Yuji Maruyama and Tatsuo Wada

*Second Department of Surgery, Faculty of Medicine, University of Tokyo, Tokyo, Japan*

Some reports have already been published on ultrasonography of carcinoma of the stomach (1-3). Almost all lesions in the literature were highly advanced Type IV of Borrmann's classification . In those reports sonography revealed diffuse thickening of the gastric wall resembling a doughnut or kidney, whereas cases with localized involvement have been reported recently (4).

To our knowledge, no report has specifically reviewed lymph node metastases of gastric cancer.

Barium and endoscopic studies are the most accurate procedures for estimating the characteristics and extent of lesions. However, serosal invasion or lymph node metastases cannot be diagnosed because these examinations observe the mucosal side. Ultrasound can delineate extragastric structures and provide information about them, because tomograms of the body can be obtained. When selecting a suitable procedure at surgery, it is important to detect serosal invasion and lymph node metastases preoperatively.

We have performed ultrasound routinely in cases with carcinoma of the stomach. In this paper we would like to report of ultrasonography and the detectability of gastric cancer and associated lymph node metastases.

MATERIALS AND METHODS

During the past five years, 154 cases of adenocarcinoma of the stomach underwent ultrasonic examination and laparotomy. Ninety-six of these had advanced cancer classified under Borrmann's classification and formed the basis of this study (Table 1). Lymph node metastases were diagnosed macroscopically at laparotomy.

These five years were divided into two periods because the resolution of the equipment improved during the latter period. Forty-three patients in the former period were scanned with conventional equipment with a focused 2.25 MHz, 19 mm trasducer. For the 53 patients in the latter period, a gray scale scanner*with a 2.25 or 3.5 MHz, 13 mm transducer and real time scanners

* Aloka SSD 120D, Aloka SSD 250 ( Aloka Co. Ltd., Tokyo)

TABLE 1. Clinical Materials

| Borrmann's | Type |
|:---|:---:|
| I | 2 |
| II | 27 |
| III | 49 |
| IV | 18 |
| Total | 96 |

(electronic linear and mechanical sector arrayed scanners) were used.

Transverse, longitudinal and right subcostal scans were obtained in fasting state. To demonstrate gastric lesions, non-sterotyped scanning was necessary. By left subcostal scan and scans made at right angles to the long axis of the stomach, the gastric wall and lymph nodes along the lesser and greater curvatures could be recognized easily. By cepharad angulation of the ultrasonic beam transverse or left subcostal scans just below the xyphoid process were able to delineate the lesser curvature of the cardia and abdominal esophagus. For this purpose sector arrayed equipment were preferred to linear arrayed ones.

The stomach was filled with 500 ml of freshly tap water, containing numerous microbubbles which produce strong echoes. The lumen of the stomach was identified definitely, because tap water exhibited a good contrast to the gastric wall which was less echogenic. The amount of water was not sufficient to fill up the stomach so that the position was changed; scanning in supine or left decubitus positon was used for lesions of the upper half of the stomach and scanning in sitting position for lesions of the antrum.

RESULTS

Gastric Tumors

Of 96 patients with advanced carcinoma, 65 cases showed thickening of the gastric wall. In twenty-six of 43 cases of the former period and 39 of 53 cases of the latter period, gastric tumors could be delineated.

There were two cases of Borrmann Type I, 76 cases of Type II or III and 18 cases of Type IV. Type I carcinoma were appeared as hypoechoic masses. Type II or III carcinomas were typically manifested as crescent or horse-shoe shapes(Fig. 1).

"Craters" could be seen when the ultrsonic beam passed through areas of ulceration (Fig. 2). This picture was enhanced by tap water in the stomach.

In sections at right angles to the long axis of the

104

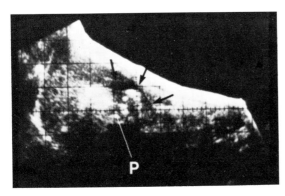

Figure 1: Borrmann Type III carcinoma is depicted(arrows).
P=pancreas

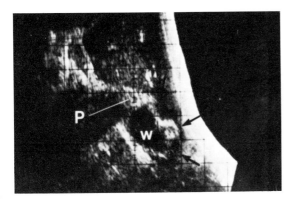

Figure 2: Crater is demonstrated. W=water in the stomach.

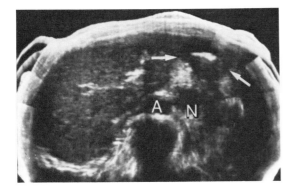

Figure 3: Borrmann Type IV carcinoma(arrows).   A=aorta,
N=lymph node metastasis.

stomach, Borrmann Type IV and far advanced Type II or III carcinomas were demonstrated as circumferential thickening of the wall, referred to as "doughnut" or "pseudokidney" shapes (Fig. 3).

Lesions occupying the cardia, principally at the lesser curvature, could be delineated in 19 out of 33 cases.

### Lymph Nodes

Lymph node metastases were depicted as round low echo areas with either conventional or gray scale equipment (Fig. 4). Larger involved nodes had irregular internal echoes. In 46 of 96 cases, metasatic lymph nodes were delineatd. Gray scale equipment exceeded conventional ones with regard to the sensitivity of detecting node involvement (Table 2). With gray scale equipment lymph node metastases were identified in 32 out of 53 cases compared to 14 out of 43 cases with conventional equipment.

The extent of lymph node metastases vary depending on the stage and occupying site of the lesions. In Japan

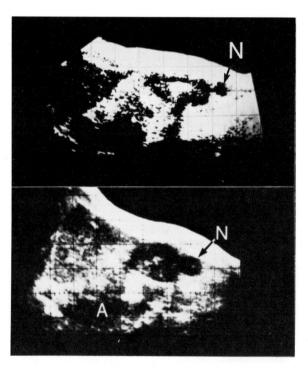

Figure 4: Lymph node metastases along the greater curvature are depicted (N). A=aorta.
Top;conventional sonogram, bottom;gray scale.

TABLE 2. Incidence of Detection of Gastric Tumors
and Lymph Node Metastases

|  | conventional | gray scale |
|---|---|---|
| No. of Cases | 43 | 53 |
| Tumor | 26 (60%) | 39 (74%) |
| Lymph Node | 14 (34%)* | 32 (60%) |

* Two cases were excluded because of no lymph
node metastasis

lymph nodes are classified clinically by the general
rules for gastric cancer, which assigns numbers for each
regional lymph node (Fig. 5). This rules evaluated the
stage of gastric cancer based of the four factors of
serosal invasion, peritoneal dissemination, and
involvement of the liver and lymph nodes. Therefore, it
is important to classify visualized lymph node according
to these rules. Since lymph nodes exist along arteries,
the celiac artery and its branches should be iedentified
for the purpose of numbering. However, small arteries,
such as the left gastric or gastroepiploic arteries, are
usually difficult to demonstrate with ultrasound.
Sometimes even thicker arteries, such as the common

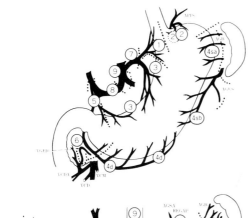

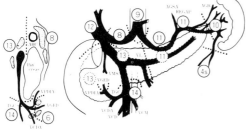

Figure 5
Lymph node classifica-
tion of the Japanese
general rules.

hepatic or splenic arteries, are difficult to delineate.
Thus accurate classification after the Japanese rules was
impossible by sonography. Some regional lymph nodes
which were adjacent to one another anatomically and after
the general rules were combined arbitrarily into several
groups. Each lymph node on sonography was classified
into the appropriate group.

Visualized lymph nodes could be accurately numbered
(Table 3). On the other hand, the sensitivity in each
group was low except for lymph nodes of the lesser
curvature or around the celiac artery where the liver
could be used as a sonic window (Table 3).

DISCUSSION

A doughnut-shaped lesion was reported as a typical
feature of neoplasms of the stomach. In our series this
characteristically represented Borrmann's Type IV
carcinoma in the antrum. Type II or III was typically
depicted as a "crescent" or "horse-shoe" shapes, when
lesions of these types were confined to a part of the
wall.

Delineation of lesions in the cardia has been
described to be difficult(5) although the opposite
opinion was recently reported (4). Our experience
indicates that this depends on the location of the
lesions and scanning technique. Lesions mainly occuping

TABLE 3.

| Lymph Node Groups | Accuracy of Numbering | | Sensitivity | |
|---|---|---|---|---|
| 1,3,5 | $\frac{27}{29}$ | (93%) | $\frac{27}{67}$ | (40%) |
| 4,6 | $\frac{14}{14}$ | (100%) | $\frac{14}{54}$ | (26%) |
| 7,8,9 | $\frac{25}{28}$ | (89%) | $\frac{25}{57}$ | (44%) |
| 10,11 | $\frac{5}{7}$ | (71%) | $\frac{5}{18}$ | (28%) |
| 12 | $\frac{3}{3}$ | (100%) | $\frac{3}{11}$ | (27%) |
| 13 | $\frac{2}{3}$ | (67%) | $\frac{2}{5}$ | (40%) |
| 16 | $\frac{5}{6}$ | (83%) | $\frac{5}{22}$ | (23%) |

the lesser curvature are easy to delineate if the ultrasodnic beam is angled cepharad and projected behind the rib cage. We encountered a patient with carcinoma of the colon in whom by delineating thickening of the lesser curvature of the cardia, cancer of the stomach was diagnosed during investigation of liver metastasis.

In one patient of the former period, sonography revealed that the lesion in the antrum eroded into the pancreas and invasion to the organ could be detected. In the latter period the transference of lesions was observed after the stomach was filled with water and posture was changed to an errect position. If the lesion and the liver or pancreas moved together, invasion was suspected. The accuracy of this method was 60%. However, as the abddominal esophagus and pyrolus are usually fixed to the diaphragm and the pancreas respectively, lesions existing around these locations would not be depart from the liver or pancreas even if there is no invasion. Therefore, further evaluation of this method are necessary although the diagnosis of serosal invasion has much clinical significance.

Involvement of paraaortic nodes were reported mainly with lymphmas. Walls (5) reported only one patient with paraaortic adenopathy, but systematic investigation of lymph node involvement in cases with gastric cancer could not be found out in the literature. In our series, 23% of paraaortic adenopathy could be detected. If involvement of paraaortic nodes is detected preoperatively, curative surgery is proved to be highly unlikely.

We think that adenopathy attainig a size of more than 1 cm can be detected although sensitivity depends on the patient's constitution and the location of lymph nodes such as those along the celiac artery. We could find out 44% of lymph node metastases around the celiac artery. If large lymph node metastases of this location are demonstrated, Appleby's procedure should be selected for en bloc resection where the celiac artery is resected at its point of divergence from the aorta.

"Spherical" swelling of lymph nodes on sonograms was considered to be metastatic. However, swelling may be due to inflamation. Some discrepancy usually exists between macroscopic and histological diagnoses of lymph node metastases. Therefore, ultrsound findings were compared with histological diagnoses. The accuracy of numbering and sensitivity showed the same tendency as those with macroscopic diagnoses.

In our study, sensitivity was low. This was partly because small metastases could no be detected by existing equipment and partly because of the location of lymph nodes. If these lymph nodes are not detected preoperatively, clinical significance is somewhat low except for paraaortic nodes, because it is easy to resect these small nodes as a mass at surgery.

REFERENCES

1. Peterson, L.R. and Cooperberg, P.L. (1978): Gastro-
   intest Radiol., 3, 303.
2. Bluth, E.T., Merritt, C.R.B. and Sullivan, M.A. (1979):
   Radiology, 133, 677.
3  Braun, W.B.S. and Dombrowski, H. (1979): J. Clin.
   Ultrasound, 7, 425
4  Yeh, H.C. and Rabinowitz, J.G. (1981): Radiology, 141
   147.
5  Walls, W.J. (1976): Radiology, 118, 159.

# ULTRASOUND IN POST-OPERATIVE FOLLOW-UP OF STOMACH AND COLONIC CARCINOMA

Wilhelm Möckel

*Innere Abteilung des Evangelischen Krankenhauses, Köln-Kalk, FRG*

In our department, ultrasonic examination using the rapid B scan has been employed routinely for the last four years as a "continuation of the clinical examination by other means" (RETTENMAIER, 1976 (3)). In 1981, 2640 patients were examined with this modality.

In these cases, the sonographic examination provided, among other things, valuable information about possible causes of upper abdominal complaints, the cause of a jaundice and, where applicable, about the localization of the obstruction and also changes to the pancreas. In patients with abdominal tumours, the pre-operative ultrasonic investigation proved useful in demonstrating or excluding the presence of liver and lymph node metastases. In two cases of carcinoma of the stomach, however, the diffuse metastatic disease within the liver was not recognized, and, indeed, the differentiation of diffuse malignant infiltration of the liver from chronic inflammatory processes with cirrhotic remodelling, is difficult (LUTZ (1)). Within the framework of the post-operative aftercare of abdominal cancers, carried out jointly with our surgical department, we have incorporated the ultrasonic investigation into the after-care programme.

## PATIENT MATERIAL AND METHODS

In 1981, within the framework of post-operative tumour after-care, 43 patients with an early gastric cancer, 3o cases of advanced gastric carcinoma and 39 patients with colo-rectal carcinomas were managed. In addition to clinical examination and a weight check, all follow-up examinations included a blood count, liver chemistry, ERS, in patients with colo-rectal carcinoma also a CEA assay-furthermore, an ultrasonic examination with the rapid B scan was performed. At fixed intervals after surgery, X-ray checks were also made of the chest, the surgically treated stomach or the colon using the double-contrast technique, alternatingly with endoscopic follow-up inspections. For ultrasonography, we employed the Vidoson 735 and the RA 1 manufactured by SIEMENS — in the last few months the Aloka SSD 256.

In general, the ultrasonic work-up comprised an examination of the entire abdomen, with special attention being paid to the surgically treated organ, the liver, the retro-peritoneal lymph nodes and also to the presence of ascites.

With respect to the contour and size of the normal liver, we oriented ourselves to the data published by WEILL (5):

Smooth, acute left-lateral and left-ventral liver edge having an angle of up to 45°,

a width of the left liver lobe of 4 cm measured from a tangent to the left edge of the vertebral body,

an angle of up to 75° at the anterior edge of the right liver lobe.

With regard to the contour of the liver, following WEILL, we differentiate physiological curvatures (beneath the edge of the costal arch in the longitudinal section, in the region of the undersurface of the liver with a promient caudate lobe, an elevation of the left lobe above the aorta in the transversal section, and beneath the lower pole of the left kidney in the longitudinal section) from humps and edge deformations that are suspicious for metastatic disease. In this connection, typical echo-poor or echogenic areas, or a combination of both representing a necrosis, occurring either solitary or multiple, subcapsular or in the depth of the parenchyma, lend support to the suspicion of metastatic disease.

While metastases were found in none of the 43 patients with surgically treated early gastric cancer over the period of observation, liver metastases were detected sonographically in five of the 30 patients subjected to surgery for advanced gastric carcinoma, 2 of these patients also having ascites. (Fig. 1 and 2).

Out of 39 patients with surgically treated colo-rectal carcinoma followed up in 1981, 7 were found to have liver metastases on sonography.

All the patients presenting with liver metastatic disease proved to have a markedly elevated alkaline phosphatase and gamma GT.

To date, no local recurrent tumour has been detected sonographically, either in surgically treated gastric carcinoma patients or in patients with colo-rectal carcinomas subjected to surgery, nor have metastases been found in retroperitoneal lymph nodes.

DISCUSSION

In the tumour after-care of our patients with surgically treated gastric carcinoma, whether early cancer or advanced cancer, and after surgical treatment for colorectal carcinomas, ultrasonography with the rapid B scan has been regularly carried out, in particular with an eye to detecting local recurrence, liver or lymph metastases.

With regard to the detection or exclusion of liver metastases, the classification proposed by LUTZ et al.(1) has proved of value:

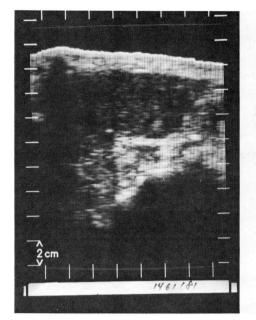

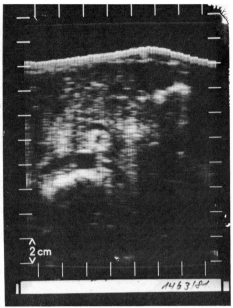

Figure 1
Metastatic hepatomegaly
Sonolucent nodules

Figure 2
Metastatic hepatomegaly
Edge sig

| | | |
|---|---|---|
| Ia | = | unremarkable liver |
| Ib | = | low-grade structural irregularities |
| IIa | = | densely structured liver |
| IIb | = | with some slight irregularities |
| III | = | inhomogeneous liver structure |
| IIIa | = | solid structural defect (s) |
| IIIb | = | irregular distribution of echoes |
| IIIc | = | cystic structural defect (s) |

   In 5 out of 30 patients with surgically-treated
advanced gastric carcinoma, and in 7 out of 39 patients
with colo-rectal carcinoma, the ultrasonic examination
revealed liver metastases, some presenting an echo-poor,
some an echo-rich (echogenic) pattern. The accumulation
found, for example, by TRILLER et al. (4), of echo-poor
metastases in gastric carcinoma, and the predominance of
echogenic foci in carcinomas of the colon, were not

113

clearly observed in our small number of cases. In all the
patients, the finding of liver metastasis was supported
by a marked elevation of alkaline phosphatase and gammaGT.
In 43 patients followed up after surgery for an early
gastric cancer, metastases have, so far, been detected
neither at sonography, nor by other investigational
modalities.

On ultrasonographic investigation of our surgical
patients with both early and advanced cancer, we have
virtually regularly found changes in the contour of the
left lobe of the liver with coarsening, roundings-off and
humps, as also structural irregularities with varyingly
large echo-poorer areas in the lateral portion of the left
lobe (2).

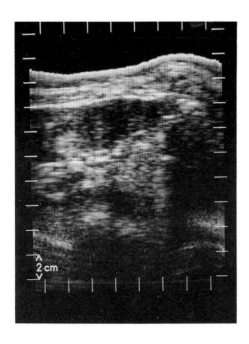

Figure 3
"Edge sign"

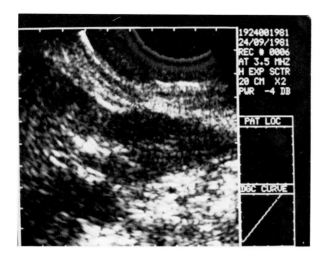

Figure 4
"Hump"

Further investigations (laparoscopy, fine-needle puncture)
and the clinical course, all excluded metastases as the
cause of these changes. These sonographically detectable
contour and structural changes of the left lobe of the
liver are apparently caused by "cords" of scar tissue
and adhesions, require a particularly careful sonographic examination and, in the presence of equivocal
findings, require a further diagnostic workup. Finally,
in patients subjected to a gastric resection, whether
for a carcinoma or an ulcer, the gastro-enteral anastomosis can usually be represented as a cockade-like structure
in close topographic relationship to the deformed left
lobe of the liver. Follow-up examinations, some of which
extended over a number of years, revealed no recognizable
changes in the anastomosis. A suspected tumour recurrence
at the anastomosis or the devolopment of a gastric stump
carcinoma in these patients was excluded endoscopically,
by sonographic follow-up studies and by the subsequent
coures.

Sonography with the rapid B scan, used on a wide scale within the internal medical department (170 beds) of a medium-sized hospital proves not only to be of use in "directing" the further diagnostic work-up in patients with unclear upper abdominal complaints, useful in the pancreatic diagnostic work-up and the therapy of obstructive jaundice, but also an important supplementary modality in the pre-operative diagnosis and post-operative aftercare of gastro-intestinal tumours.

REFERENCES

1.    Lutz, H., Reichel, L., Heyder, N., Ehler, R., Petzold, R. (1980): In: Ultraschalldiagnostik in der Medizin, p. 101
      Editors: M. Hinselmann, M. Anliker and R. Mendt.
      Georg Thieme, Stuttgart - New York.

2.    Möckel, W., Schmidt, W. and Hornung, Chr.: Über Ultraschallbefunde der Leber nach Magenresektion (1981): In Press.

3.    Rettenmaier, G. (1976): Internist, 17, 549.

4.    Triller, J., Fuchs, W.A. (1980):
      Abdominale Sonographie
      Georg Thieme, Stuttgart - New York.

5.    Weill, F.S. (1978):
      Ultrasonography of Digestive Diseases
      The C.V. Mosby Company, St. Louis.

# DIAGNOSIS OF HEPATIC METASTASIS. ANATOMOECHOGRAPHIC CORRELATIONS ABOUT 111 CASES

M.Ch. Plainfosse, Ph. Bor and J.P. Delalande

*Department of Echography and Radiology, Broussais Hospital, Paris, France*

After discovering a neoplasic disease the study of the liver for secondary localizations is necessary to assess its extension and to control it after treatment,(3) The positivity of this research determines the therapeutic strategy and prognosis.

The reliability, safety and cheap cost of echotomography makes it a very good technique to study the liver.

We have compared the results obtained by echotomography with the data of manual exploration by the surgeon (101 cases) or laparoscopy (10 cases).

## MATERIALS AND METHODS

111 patients, 64 males and 47 females, with known neoplasic localizations went through an echotomographic exam, looking for secondary hepatic impairment before operation or laparoscopic verification.

Echographic equipment included a real-time instrument Combison 100 Kretz with a 2,25 MHz transducer including five transmitter-receivers crystals rotating and focussed at different depths, and a manual B-mode echograph Sonia CGR with 2,25 MHz, 3,5 MHz and 5 MHz transducers.

Echographic sections were made according to four principal axes : sagittal, transverse recurrent subcostal, oblique recurrent subcostal and intercostal. The whole hepatic parenchyma was studied according to these different axes, several times during the same exam. Gallbladder intra and extra hepatic biliary ducts, portal vein, supra-hepatic veins, inferior vena cava, pancreas, right diaphragmatic pleura were studied simultaneously.

The global size of the liver was estimated and measured at the nipple line and at the epigastrium. The sharp angle of the inferior boundary of the liver was often blunted when it was enlarged because of the secondary localizations.

The visualization of an evocative aspect of metastasis according to two different axes in the same hepatic segment justifies the diagnosis of secondary localization.

The hepatic segmentation is based upon the supra

hepatic veins distribution. The accurate localization of the hepatic masses was often difficult because several segments were often impaired by the same mass.

RESULTS

The following table summarizes our study :

| M 64<br>F 47 = 111 | ECHOGRAPHY | SURGERY OR<br>LAPAROSCOPY |
| --- | --- | --- |
| Liver + | 32 | 24 +<br>8 - |
| Liver - | 75 | 2 +<br>73 - |
| Doubtful | 4 | 1 +<br>3 - |

+ with metastasis
- without metastasis

Out of 107 expressed diagnoses, 97 were corroborated by the  surgical exploration or laparoscopy (90,6 %)

The false positives were 8 out of 32 patients. The specificity was therefore 75 %. But among these 8 false positives we found : one infected biliary cyst, one liver cell adenoma, one hepatic abscess.

Their echographic aspect, associated with carcinologic history was not distinguishable from liver metastasis aspects. If we take this into account, the specificity of the echographic diagnosis in the detection of pathological intra hepatic masses rises to 84,3 %.

The others false positives (5 out of 8) were cirrhotic liver with fibrosis and regenerative nodules.

The false negatives were due to the small size of the metastasis, less than 2 cm.

Paradoxycally, the broad size of some hepatic tumors the strusture and density of which were not much different from the contiguous parenchyma could make the diagnosis difficult. This is true in particular for the hepatomas which the computed tomography diagnosis failed to find in 20 % of cases with the first generation equipment. (1)

## DISCUSSION

About the diagnosis of intrahepatic masses the different papers on this subject give an accuracy of :
a) 72 % (5) to 90 % (22) with echography
b) 68 % to 90 %  with radionuclid imaging (21)
c) 88 % (6) to 96 % (7) with computed tomography.

With an accuracy of 90,6 % our study indicates that the diagnosis with echography improves with the experience of the operator and the amelioration of the equipment. We checked the particular reliability of our real-time equipment for the diagnosis of hepatic metastasis with other authors.

The smallest hepatic tumors diagnosed with echography measured about 2 cm in diameter. 37 % were more than 4 cm (20). The largest ones could be over 12 cm in diameter. The metastases were alone in 30 % of cases, dual in 16 %, multiple in 64 % of cases (23).

The hepatic metastasis could appear with various echographic aspects classified according to their density compared to the normal hepatic parenchyma (9,11,12,14 20,23).
- increased density : 30 %
- decreased density : 18 to 23 %
- association of both : 10 % to 17 %
- calcified : 3 %
- partly or in totality liquid : 4 %

The others aspects showed zones of mixed density without a clear boundary with an infiltrating and anarchic aspect. "Bull eye" aspect is rather characteristic of hepatic metastasis (14). The echographic imaging showed a dense mass with a less dense blurring due to congestive sinusoïd vessels surrounding the dense mass. This aspect would be present in 17 % of cases (20).

A transonic mass is not obligatorily liquid. A-mod is interesting to assert the liquid nature of certain masses. In mixed masses the liquid zone is surrounded by a thick and irregular wall. A posterior enhancement behind the mass varies in intensity from a lesion to another in the same patient. This enhancement is often very tiny if the mass is not liquid (22,23). The histological nature of the metastatic mass cannot be reliably determined by echography.(9)

Unfortunately no histological correlations could be made, so only a statical frequency can give a low probability :
- adenocarcinoma especially from the colon would more often show high density aspects and more often enclose calcifications (11,18)
- lymphomas, sarcomas and Hodgkin disease would show transonic aspects (7,8,21)

The differential diagnosis of the hepatic anomalies discovered by echography is made :

1 ) with primary tumors : hepatomas and adenomas
(2,10,11,17) :
   a) the echographic aspect of hepatomas is not specific. The diagnosis can only be surmised with the clinical
context. In a context of cirrhosis, chronic hepatitis,
syphilis or of coloured people (10) an echographic anarchic structure or the presence of dense hepatic masses
evokes the diagnosis. But invading tumors can be isodense  to the adjacent parenchyma. The false negatives
vary from 12 % (17) to 28 % (5). The computed tomography
can fail from 4 % (17) to 21 % (5,13). The same aspects
can be shown by metastasis, cirrhosis, steatosis, hemo-
chromatosis or lymphoma (11). In this case the radionuclid imaging seems more regularly positive but a metastasis can be mistaken for an abscess (10,15,18)
   b) among benign hepatic tumors, the adenomas seem
more frequent. The adenomas are distinguished from the
focal hyperplasias by containing neither Kuppfer cells
nor biliary ducts, yet there is no echographic difference. They show transonic masses sometimes with liquid
hemorragic or necrotic zones with hepatomegaly. An oestro-
genic or obesity context is sometimes found (19).
Necrotic metastases, abscesses, hemangiomas can show
some similar aspects. Yet, the association of an echographic mass with a normal radionuclid imaging would
suggest the diagnosis of adenoma.
2) with non tumoral hepatic liquid collections :
the polycystic disease is easily recognised by the association of multiple liquid masses in the liver, the
kidneys and sometimes in the pancreas.
The hepatic solitary cyst can be sometimes discriminated
with difficulty from a necrotic or hemorragic metastasis,
especially if this cyst is infected (one case in our
series).
The hepatic abscess shows an echographic aspect of a
liquid mass containing some echoes. Its wall is thick
and irregular with tiny enhancement.
The clinical context is evocative. The acute necrosis
of an hepatic tumor can mimick it (one case in our series)
Multiple micro abscesses spread in the liver can make
numerous little liquid masses in a parenchyma the structure of which is altered by dense fibrous and inflammatory zones.
   A hepatic hematoma under the Glisson's capsula or
within the parenchyma occurs in a traumatic or iatro-
genic context. Its various and evolutive aspects will be
surveyed by echography.
   Hydatic cysts show liquid masses with thick wall
sometimes calcified and septated. If a flotting membrane
is seen, it is the best symptom in favour of hydatidosis.
3) with a diffuse hepatic infiltration :
   - steatosis give a diffuse enhancement of the density
which approaches the diaphragmatic density (22). There

is a clinical context of plethoric, alcoholism or obesity.
- amyloïdis shows a near aspect,
- cirrhosis increases the density which is irregular
- acute hepatitis shows an inflammatory syndrom which magnifies the echogenicity,
- lymphoïd infiltrations can be homogeneous or heterogeneous.

CONCLUSION :

The echotomography is a very accurate technique for the diagnosis and surveillance of pathological hepatic masses. Its accessibility and its cheap cost associated with its lack of irradiation makes echography an easily repetitive exam.
   Its performances can still be increased by percutaneous biopsy directed by echography (4) or per-operation examination (16) with high frequency transducer increasing the resolution  : this allows a more accurate diagnosis of masses smaller in diameter.

REFERENCES

1.  Alfidi R., Haaga J., Havrilla R., Pepe R., Cook S., (1976) : AJR.  127 : 69-74.
2.  Angres G., Carter J.B., Velasco J.M., (1980) AJR. 135 : 172.
3.  Bernardino M.E., Green B., (1979): Radiology. 133 : 437.
4.  Bret P.M., Fond A., Labadie M., Bretagnolle M., Bret P. (1981) : RSNA. Chicago. 342 - 200.
5.  Broderick T.W., Gosink B., Mannack L., Harris R., Wilcox J. (1980) : Radiology. 135 : 149.
6.  Bryan P.J., Dinn W.N., Gronman Z.D., Wistow B.W., Mac Afee J.G., Kieffer S.A. (1977) : Radiology 124 : 387 - 393.
7.  Felix E.L., Bagley D.H., Sindelar W.F., Johnston G.S. Ketlham A.S. (1977) : Radiology 123 : 834.
8.  Ginaldi S., Bernardino M.E., Jing Bad S., Green B., (1980) Radiology 136 : 427.
9.  Green B., Bree R.L., Goldstein H.M., Stanley C. (1977) Radiology 124 : 203.
10. Hillman B.J., Smith E.H., Gammelgaard S., Holen H.H. (1980) : Radiology 135 : 269.
11. Kamin P.D., Bernardino M.E., Green B. (1979) Radiology 131 : 459.
12. Katragadda L.S., Goldstein H.M., Green B. (1979) AJR. 129 : 591.
13. Kawasaki H., Sakagushi S., Toshitake I. (1978) Am. J. Gastroenterol. 69 : 436 - 442.
14. Laval-Jeantet M., Vadrot D., Bouzac H., Buy J.N. (1980) J. Radiol. 61 : 548.

15. Mac Ardle C.R. (1976) J. Clin. Ultrasound.
    4 : 265 - 268.
16. Merran S., Plainfossé M.C. (1981) RSNA. Chicago
    98 : 119.
17. Passail G., Lacaine F., Couanet D., Piekarski J.D.,
    Kunstlinger F., Vawel D., Masselot J. (1980)
    J. Radiol. 61,11 : 655 - 659
18. Petasnik J.P., Ram P., Turner D.A., Fordham E.W.
    (1979) SNM. 9 : 8.
19. Sandler M.A., Petrocelli R.D., Marks D.S.,
    Lopez R. (1980) Radiology 135 : 393
20. Scheible W., Gosink B., Leopold G.R. (1977)
    AJR. 129 : 983.
21. Snow J.H., Goldstein H.M., Wallace S. (1979)
    AJR. 132 : 915.
22. Taylor K.H.W., Carpenter D.A., Hill C.R. (1976)
    Radiology 119 : 415 - 423.
23. Wooten W.B., Green B., Goldstein H.M. (1978)
    Radiology 128 : 447 - 450.

# ULTRASONIC EVALUATION AND THE TISSUE CHARACTERIZATION OF LIVER METASTASES: DIAGNOSIS AND THERAPEUTIC EVALUATION

Walter-L. Curati and Brigitte Curati-Nicca

*Diagnostic Radiology Department and Oncologic Center, University Hospital of Geneva, Geneva, Switzerland*

## INTRODUCTION

Gray-scale ultrasound has been greatly improved by digital processing of pictures with the aid of a small computer. Since the beginning of medical ultrasonography, the evaluation of echo-amplitude in diffuse and focal disease has been accomplished by means of :
a) A-Mode analysis, and       b) B-Scan studies
B-Scan analysis is performed in a specific area of an organ but also can be compared with adjacent regions on the same scanning picture.

Since 1977 several programs of image processing have been under study for research purposes or simpler ones for clinical use. Since 1978 we have been using such a computerized analysis with an ultrasound machine using a digital format. One of our research programs was developped in cooperation with the oncologists for the study of liver metastases.

## PATIENTS AND METHODS

We presently perform follow-ups on 300 patients presenting with liver metastases. The average period of study is 18 months. This is due to the fact that applying this method from 1978 on and including all types of liver metastases we must consider :
a) the death rate due to the primary neoplasm, and
b) the adjunction of more patients during this period
We think that such a clinical research project should have two aims   :
1. Follow-up of liver metastases for patients who have been or are currently under chemotherapy.
2. Tissue characterization of new patients : all those who have echographic evidence of abnormality first discovered by ultrasound or by nuclear medicine after clinical examination or conventional X-Ray study. Additional patients who have been first studied by Body CT are also included in the case of ultrasonic eva-

luation of therapeutic response in metastases.

Computerized analysis is commercialy available in ultrasound imaging machines using the digital format (Siemens-PHO-Sonic B-Scanner). The computer allows to study a region of interest (which should be of the same format in order to compare two adjacent regions) and displays a histogram of echo-intensity. Comparisons are easily made on the same scan for adjacent areas. It must be also emphasized that the areas of interest should be selected at the same depth from the skin surface in order to obtain the same attenuation due to the characteristics of the considered transducer (focal length) and curve settings on the A-Scan. In that way we think that it is possible to avoid as many errors as possible. Only single sweeps should be analyzed also with the same scanning speed : in such a way we will avoid other mis-reading due to overfilling or underfilling of the matrics of the digital scan converter.

The histograms produced in our machine display the relative number of echoes of a given intensity on the Y-axis and the varying levels of intensity are plotted on the X-axis. In comparing a region of interest with a so-called "normal" area we can evaluate as safely as possible two regions for their relative echogenicity.

The liver

Many situations are to be considered :
A - Metastases : focal (nodular) or diffuse
B - Metabolic changes :
- alteration of echogenicity due to chemotherapy without metastatic involvement of the liver
- diffuse non neoplastic diseases : fatty infiltration, cirrhosis, hemosiderosis, collagen-diseases, etc.

Metastatic liver

Our specific clinical application shows that size reductions or central necrosis of metastases in patients under chemotherapy are very well demonstrated by means of Computerized Image Processing (CIP). We have performed an average of 3 examinations per patient. At the beginning of our study in 1978 we used to compare every first examination with a nuclear medicine investigation or a Body CT. Since mid-1980, the clinicians don't any more ask nuclear medicine or computerized tomography for this precise application. It is now established that sensitivity is slightly higher in ultrasound than in nuclear medicine and that specificity is of course much higher in ultrasound. Comparing ultrasound and Body CT it must be said that in

the case of isoechogenic metastases sensitivity of ultrasound is lower than Body CT. On the other hand it is well
known that isodense metastases are not seen in Body CT
except if routine contrast injection is performed. In the
case of Body CT the degree of sensitivity is also closely
related with : a) the thickness of the slice, and b) the
number of slices ("one-step" or "two-step").

RESULTS

Introducing the aspect of histograms we will first
show 3 cases of diffuse liver disease :
 a)  Right heart failure with hypoechogenic liver :
     71 years old lady presenting with severe right heart
     failure : the area of interest in the middle of the
     right lobe of the liver shows a "single peak" of low
     density echoes.
 b)  Liver cirrhosis : ascitis and irregular contours of
     the liver are clearly seen on this longitudinal B-
     Scan. The region of interest is located in the mid-
     dle of the right lobe of the liver and the histogram
     shows an enlarged peak of moderate echo intensity.
     The next example will show that it is not possible
     to make an absolute difference between cirrhosis and
     fatty liver : several studies have shown that there
     is no statistic relationship between these two disea-
     ses. This case b) corresponds to a 36 years old man
     presenting with a severe alcoholic disease and cir-
     rhosis. This diagnosis was confirmed by liver biopsy
     performed under ultrasonic control.

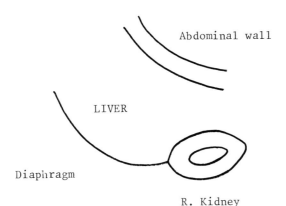

R. Kidney

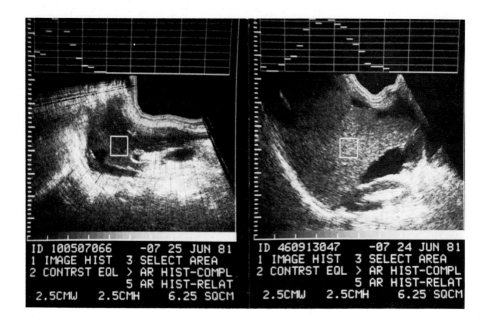

Fig. 1    a) R heart failure          b) cirrhosis

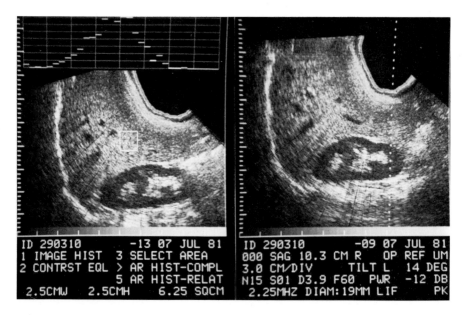

Fig. 2    Steatosis

c) Diffuse fatty infiltration : the french literature describes this aspect as "foie brillant" showing clearly the brightness of the picture. A slightly irregular peak with irregular slopes too is seen on this histogram.

Six cases of metastatic disease of the liver will be presented :

I - This 48 years old lady presented one year ago an adenocarcinoma of the large bowel. The sonogram performed then showed no evidence of metastatic involvement of the liver. One year later she presents with a severe weight loss and abdominal tenderness. The ultrasound clearly demonstrates multiple metastases in the liver and on the peritoneum. Ascitis is also present. The picture shows a specimen of metastases on the peritoneum and on the right hand an area inside the liver demonstrates the abnormality of echo density mainly due to the interposition of a bowel loop between the liver and the peritoneum. In this case we are not allowed to compare any region of "standard" liver.

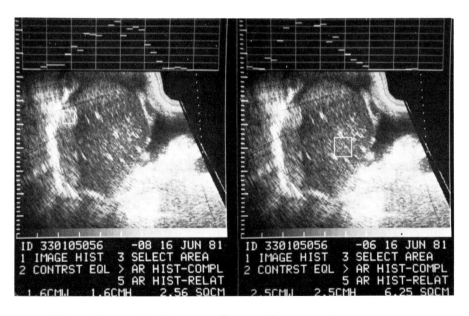

Fig. I : metastases of an adenocarcinoma

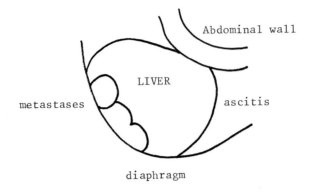

II - This 66 years old lady presented two years ago with an adenocarcinoma of the signoid. On the CT, ultrasound and nuclear medicine investigations were performed and showed no evidence of liver involvement. She now presents with multiple nodular elements showing an hypoechogenic curve which is also very irregular. On the right hand picture we can read the anatomical references and the curve settings (TGC and attenuation settings) as well as the type of transducer used for that application.

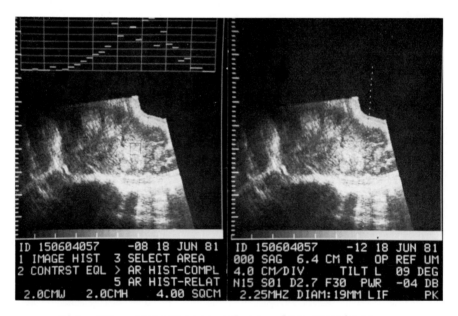

Fig. II : metastases of an adenocarcinoma

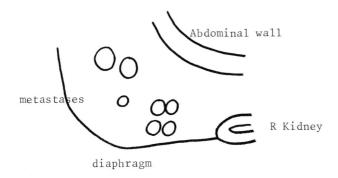

Abdominal wall

metastases

R Kidney

diaphragm

III - This 69 years old lady presents with a large
ulcerated carcinoma of the breast. The ultrasound examination reveals areas of hypoechogenicity due to the con-
fluence of several metastatic foci.

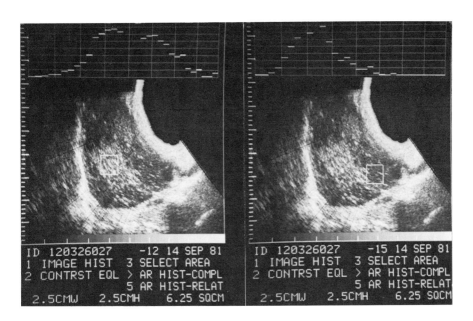

Fig. III : metastases of a carcinoma of the breast

IV - This 60 years old gentleman presents with a carcinoma of the stomach. The ultrasound of the liver shows multiple nodular areas of hyper- and also hypoechogenicity : the larger metastases are very inhomogeneous which corresponds to areas of necrosis in the masses. This can also be seen in the case of chemotherapy.

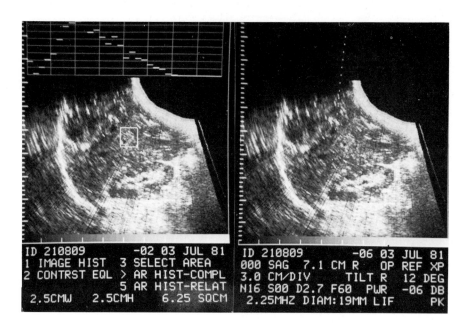

Fig. IV : metastases of a carcinoma of the stomach

V - This 57 years old lady presented 4 years ago a carcinoma of the breast. She went under radical mastectomy and, one year later, was treated with chemotherapy for the appearance of liver metastases. Two years later the ultrasound clearly shows nodular very-hypoechogenic masses in the liver. A shadowing effect is seen distally to these densities. The former presence in this region of larger metastases and secondly the shadowing effect leads to the diagnosis of calcified metastases after chemotherapy. In this case we performed additional Body CT which confirmed our diagnosis.

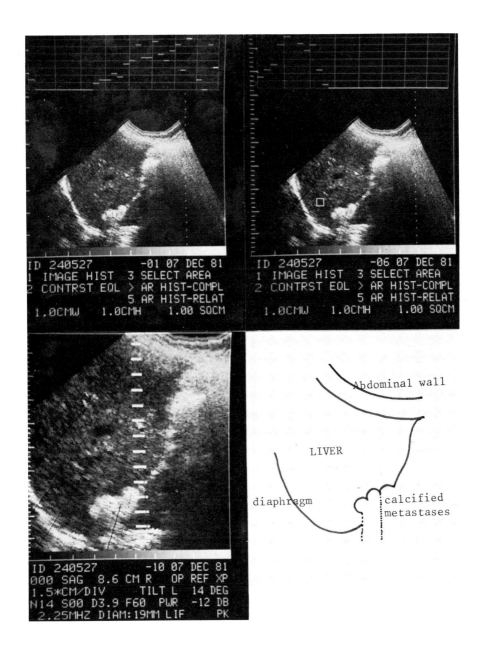

Fig. V : calcification of metastases after chemotherapy

VI - 61 years old lady presenting with epigastric pain, nausea and vomiting. An ultrasound examination has been performed immediately and reveals first a severe thickening of the gastric walls and secondly multiple metastases in the liver : the so called "cocarde" appearance in the french literature revealing metastases of sarcomatous origin opposed to the carcinomatous appearance. Gastroscopy and biopsy reveals a sarcoma of the stomach. The "en cocarde" appearance is due to the rapid growth of the metastases and the edema of the surrounding liver. As a curiousity the right hand picture showing both liver and kidney reveals a double kidney with two distinct excretory systems.

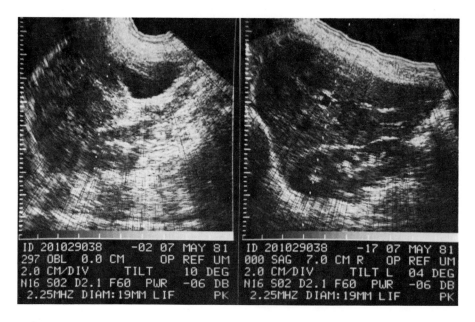

Fig. VI : metastatic involvement of the liver

In case of this "target" appearance of the metastases it seems useless to perform an histogram of the tissue, at least when these "targets" are of a small size : this is due to the fact that the tissues sampling for the histogram would be to small to be of any statistical value. This is also the case for very large masses with quite different appearances.

Area selections and measurements are not only used in order to allow a precise histogram but also in order to mesure differences in volumes of metastases during a long-term follow-up. The study of metastatic growth has been described as a biological process corresponding better to the Gompertz equation than the exponential growth. That means that a specific growth rate declines as the metastases enlarge. On the other side, with exponential growth the growth rate is constant. In our application for the assessment of a therapeutic success due to chemotherapy we can see that the Gompertzial growth is not any more a linear decrease of the growth rate referring to time but a down ward deviation of the curve representing mathematically the response to therapy.

For that precise application ultrasound is much more useful than Body CT due to the possibility of "slicing" the liver not only in transverse section (or longitudinal and frontal reconstructions).

CONCLUSIONS

On a large group of patients ultrasound has demonstrated to be a very useful diagnostic modality as well as a valuable tool for evaluation of chemotherapy.

300 patients and 1000 examinations allow us to show the high value of sensitivity and specificity of ultrasound in the assessment of liver metastases.

Being non-invasive and non-expensive (compared mainly with Body CT) ultrasonography is an ideal tool for making follow-ups.

The combined use of high-resolution real-time ultrasonography and computerized assisted B-Scanning seem to be the best combination for the 1982 sonographer.

REFERENCES

1. Birnholtz J.C. (1979) In : Ultrasound in Gastrointestinal Disease. Clinics in Diagnostic Ultrasound 1. p. 23-34, Editors : Taylor K.J.W., Churchill Livingstone, New York.
2. Curati W.L., Curati-Nicca B., Alberto P., Wettstein P. (1981) : NBS Publications, US Dept of Commerce, Gaithersburg, Maryland, USA.
3. Jaffe C.C., Taylor K.J.W. (1979) : Radiology 131, 469.
4. Taylor K.J.W., Gorelick F.S., Rosenfield A.T. et al. (1981) : Radiology 141, 157-161.
5. Weill F.S. (1979) : Ultrasonography of Digestive Diseases, Mosby.

# THE DIAGNOSIS OF GALLBLADDER CARCINOMA WITH ULTRASOUND IMAGE

Yoshikazu Yasuda[1], Akiyoshi Kashii[1], Kogoro Kasahara[1] and Kouichi Itoh[2]

[1]*Department of Surgery and* [2]*Department of Clinical Pathology, Jichi Medical School, Japan*

Ultrasonography is highly accurate in diagnosing gallbladder diseases. The diagnosis of gallbladder carcinoma is still difficult in the early stages. In order to evaluate the usefulness of ultrasonography in the diagnosis of gallbladder carcinoma, the authors reviewed 24 such cases (17 female, 7 male) during the period 1976 to 1982.

| Type | | No.of Cases | Resection | |
|:---:|:---:|:---:|:---:|:---:|
| | | | Curative | non-Curative |
| **I** | | I | I | 0 |
| **II** | | 6 | 5 | I |
| **III** | | 6 | I | 4 |
| **IV** | | 7 | 0 | 0 |

Type I: Fungating mass on the gallbladder wall like a polyp; Type II: fungating mass with partially thickened wall; Type III: gallbladder wall totally thickened with or without partially fungation; Type IV: gallbladder filled with mass. ST(+); HINF(+); H(+); B(+); N(+); HINF(susp); H(susp); B(susp); N(susp); ST(-); HINF(-); H(-); B(-); N(-). (ST: stone; HINF: hepatic infiltration; H: liver metastasis; B: bile duct infiltration; N: lymph node metastasis.)

Gallbladder carcinoma was correctly diagnosed in 20 patients by ultrasonic image. Our diagnostic accuracy was 83% by only ultrasonic findings and there were some cases which could not be differentiated from ohter benign or malignant lesions.

We classified gallbladder carcinoma in 4 types by ultrasonic image modifying Yeh's classification. One case was a fungating mass like a polyp (Type I), 6 cases were fungating mass with partially thickened wall (Type II), 6 had totally thickened wall with partial fungation (Type III), and 7 had gallbladder filled with mass (Type IV). Carcinoma of Type I or II could be resected curatively, but most cancers of Type IV could not be removed or operated in this study.

Recently, for confirming the diagnosis we used aspiration biopsy under ultrasonic guidance to the tumor and bile juice in the gallbladder. Our 7 patients were subjected to needle aspiration biopsy. The cytological study of gallbladder carcinoma was highly accurate and there were no false-positives and false-negatives. At the same time, radiographic visualization of the gallbladder was obtained by injecting contrast medium through the needle. Radiography of the gallbladder yields some beneficial findings for diagnosis and surgery. It shows the infiltration of carcinoma to the bile duct which is not detected by ultrasonography.

# RADIAL SCAN ULTRASONOGRAPHY FOR ESTIMATING THE EXTENSION OF THE CERVICAL CARCINOMA

Kaoru Sekiba, Nobuo Akamatsu, Akira Yuhara, Akinori Obata and Satoru Fukumoto

*Department of Obstetrics and Gynecology, Okayama University Medical School, Okayama, Japan*

Estimating the extension of cervical carcinoma outside the uterus has traditionally been done by bimanual
and rectal examinations with the assistance of colposcopic
examination or intravenous pyelography. Bimanual and rectal examinations, however, largely rely upon the phisi-
cian's intuition and experience. Because of this, those
examinations lack objectivity. Cystoscopic examination and
intravenous pyelography are the methods effectively used
only when the cancer has widely spread. On the other hand,
the body imaging method in diagnosing has improved remarkably, and recently has been used in determinating the
spread of cervical cancer. We, in addition, are applying
ultrasonography(USG) in this field. This paper describes
the radial scan method and how to read the images displayed and the results.

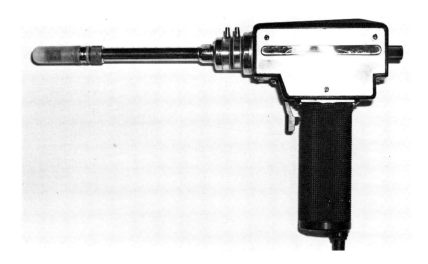

Figure 1. Probe for transrectal radial scanning, 15 mm in
diameter

Preparatory treatment is intestinal irrigation to get rid of masses feces in the rectum, full bladder technique for marking, and insertion of water balloon into the posterior fornix of the vagina. After covering a probe(Figure 1) with a rubber sac, it is inserted into the rectum and 100 ml of water is filled inbetween the probe and the rubber sac(1). When the tomographic image is displayed on the cathod ray tube(CRT), and parametrium is observed dierctly cephalad the water balloon in the posterior fornix of the vagina(Figure 2). Normal parametrium should be displayed on the CRT as a strip with low amplitude, whereas parametrial induration causes changes in length, width, and echo amplitude. The degree of parametrial induration estimated by rectal examination and at laparotomy is classified, in our department, into following five classes; 1) Not indurated:(-), 2)Slightly indurated:(+), 3)Moderately indurated:(卄), 4)Moderate-severely indurated:(卅), and 5) Indurated to the pelvic wall:(卌).

In 68 cases radical hysterectomy for cervical cancer (FIGO stage I:33 cases, II:35 cases) was performed from February, 1980 to June, 1981. We studied 136 paramatria observed in both sides of the cervix by transrectal radial scan USG about the length, width, the product of

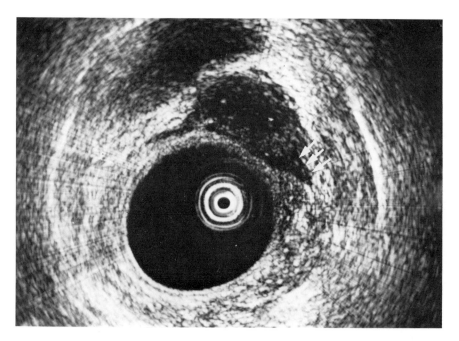

Figure 2. Echogram obtained by transrectal radial scanning shows left thickened parametrium(arrow).

the two and amplitude of the parametrial echo. Figure 3-5 and Table 1 show the results of the estimation of these changes compared with the diagnosis of parametrial induration palpated at the operation(2). As stage Ⅲ was not included in the 68 cases who were performed radical or modified radical hysterectomies, parametrial induration on class (╫) was also not found, needless to say. A statistically significant difference between the group of para-

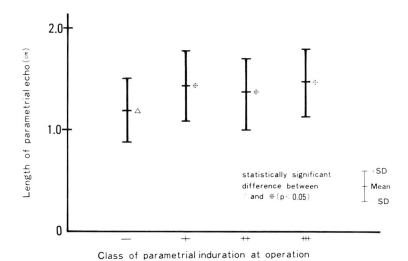

Figure 3. Correlation between class of parametrial induration and length of parametrial echo

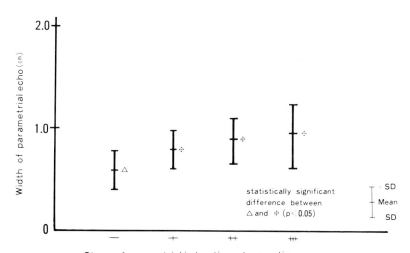

Figure 4. Correlation between class of parametrial induration and width of parametrial echo

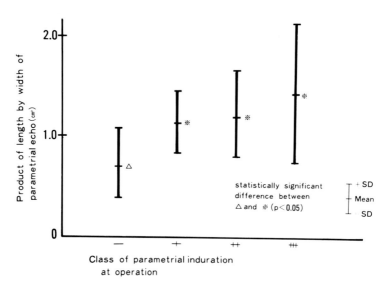

Figure 5. Correlation between class of parametrial induration and product of length by width of parametrial echo

Table 1. Correlation between class of parametrial induration and amplitude of parametrial echo

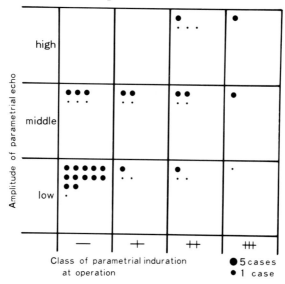

metrial induration(-) and each group of (+), (++) and (+++)
was recognized by Student's t test, in studying the length,
width and the product of the two in parametrial echo. However, a significant difference among parametrial indura-
tion(+), (++) and (+++) was not recognized. The relationship between the degree of echo amplitude and parametrial

140

Table 2. Correlation between more induration side of parametria and shift of cervix on echogram

**More indurative side at operation**

echo there is, a fact considered significant by chi-squere
test. It was also obserevd that more uterine cervix was
displayed on the more indurated side(Table 2)(2).

In order to estimate the effectiveness of radiotherapy for cervical carcinoma, we carries it out for 7
cases of FIGO stage IIb, 23 cases of stage IIIb and 2 cases
of stage IV(3). Table 3 shows the changes of the length,
width and the product of the two in parametrial echo at
the moment before therapy, mid-point of therapy(mean radiation doses of point B:3550 rad) and after therapy(mean
radiation doses of point B:7080 rad). They are significantly different respectively.

Table 3. Changes of length, width and product of the two
in parametrial echo during the radiotherapy

|  | Length (Mean ± SD) | Width (Mean ± SD) | Product (Mean ± SD) |
|---|---|---|---|
| Before Therapy | 1.48 ± 0.25 | 0.91 ± 0.22 | 1.37 ± 0.46 |
| Mid-point of Therapy | 1.33 ± 0.26* | 0.85 ± 0.23 | 1.15 ± 0.42* |
| After Therapy | 1.23 ± 0.23* | 0.74 ± 0.23* | 0.93 ± 0.32* |

SD:standard deviation
* :significantly different values compared with the value
before therapy by Student's t test(P 0.05)

TRANSURETHRAL INTRAVESICAL RADIAL SCAN USG FOR ESTIMATING
VESICAL INFILTRATION OF CERVICAL CARCINOMA

A study in order to estimate the degree of muscular
infiltration in carcinoma of the urinary bladder was conducted with the transurethral intravesical radial scan
method. It was reported that a tumor with marked thickness
was observed on the bladder wall, or that a rather sonolucent mass occupied the whole thickened wall and interrupted the normal wall with strong echoes(4).

A systematic study concerning the bladder echo pattern on metastasis of the cervical cancer has not been reported. The bladder wall and the uterine cervix are observed, using a fine probe(7 mm in diameter) showed in
Figure 6, in order to diagnose the extension of cervical
cancer to the urinary bladder. Twenty-seven cases of cervical carcinoma were performed the transurethral radial
scanning during the period from February, 1980 to October,
1981. Those cases consisted of 7 FIGO stage Ⅱ cervical
cancer cases, 16 stage Ⅲ cases and 4 stage Ⅳ cases(Table
4) (5). A thin smooth two-layers echo pattern, considered to indicate normal bladder wall was observed in the 13
cases(Figure 7). No abnormality was seen any of those
cases by cystoscopic examination. In 4 cases showed thick
two-layers structure, likewise, abnormality of the bladder
was not observed cystoscopically. There were two cases
showing an irregular outer layer with a smooth inner layer,
but no cancerous infiltration by cystoscopic examination.
However, the change in the serous membrane or in the muscular couldn't be observed because laparotomy was not per-

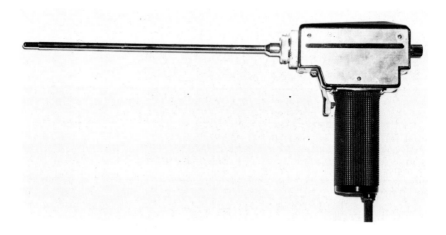

Figure 6. Probe for transurethral intravesical radial
scanning, 7 mm in diameter

Table 4. Correlation between type of echo pattern of urinary bladder and FIGO staging of cervical carcinoma and cystoscopical cancer invasion

| Type of Echo Pattern | FIGO Stage | | | | Cystoscopical Bladder Invasion | | No. of Cases |
|---|---|---|---|---|---|---|---|
| | I | II | III | IV | (−) | (+) | |
| Thin Smooth Two-layers Structure | 0 | 5 | 8 | 0 | 13 | 0 | 13 |
| Thick Smooth Two-layers Structure | 0 | 2 | 2 | 0 | 4 | 0 | 4 |
| Structure with De-stroyed One Layer | 0 | 0 | 2 | 0 | 2 | 0 | 2 |
| Structure with De-stroyed Two Layers | 0 | 0 | 4 | 4 | 1 | 7 | 8 |
| Total | 0 | 7 | 16 | 4 | 20 | 7 | 27 |

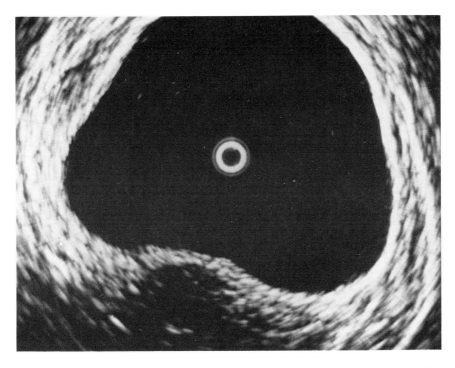

Figure 7. Thin two-layers structure of urinary bladder——
No cervical cancer invasion to urinary bladder

formed for these two cases. There were eight cases where
the two-layers structure in the bladder wall was destroyed
and made irregular, with seven cases in which the metastatic cancer were observed cystoscopically(Figure 8). The
rest one, which was a reccurent case, has formed pyometra
together with a cervical myoma adhered to the bladder. The
application of transurethral intravesical radial scan USG
to the estimation of infiltrated cervical carcinoma to the
urinary bladder has just started, besides, the bladder is
the region where biopsy is not easily performed because of
bleeding after biopsy, so results obtained by USG are hard
to compare with the obtained by histological examination.
Nevertheless, the boundary layer between the mucosa and
the myometrium, and the boundary between the muscle and
the serosa or surrounding tissue of the bladder show echogenic, the inside of the myometrium shows echo poor, so
they shows two-layers echogenic linear echo pattern. Therefore, if cervical carcinoma spreads from outer surface of
the serosa to the myometrium, the outer layer shows irregularity or is destroyed. Moreover, if it infiltrates all
the myometrium, both layers can be destroyed. Ultimately,
it seems to be recognized as a mass protruded from the

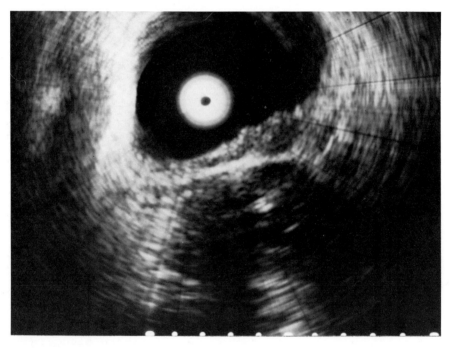

Figure 8. Destroyed two-layers structure and mass formation——Cervical cancer metastasis to urinary bladder

mucous membrane surface.

These conditions can be observed by the transabdominal USG, but the transurethral intravesical radial scannig, at which an irradiated ultrasound beam with a short wavelength and good resolvability from a short distance is utilized, has fulfilled expectations. Compared with X-ray computed tomography, radial scan USG has some real advantage, because it is inexpensive, and requires no special room. Along with the further improvement of the device, images with better resolution have been improving. Therefore, it seems to be considered that the transrectal and transurethral radial scan USG are widely used. there is increasing necessity or an objective and consistent image diagnosis to quickly curb the extension of cervical cancer.

REFERENCES

1. Sekiba, K., Fujita, T., Akamatsu, N., Obata, A., Fukumoto, S., Goto, R., Hirai, T., Kawai, J. and Niwa, K. (1980): JSUM Proceedings, 36, 213.
2. Sekiba, K., Yuhara, A., Akamatsu, N., Obata, A., Fukumoto, S., Kawai, J., Hirai, T., Niwa, K. and Nishi, M. (1981): JSUM Proceedings, 39, 101.
3. Sekiba, K., Yuhara, A., Akamatsu, N., Obata, A., Fukumoto, S., Hirai, T., Kawai, J., Fujita, T. and Niwa, K.(1982): JSUM Proceedings, 40, in press.
4. Nakamura, S., Niijima, T. (1980): J. Urology, 124, 341.
5. Sekiba, K., Akamatsu, N., Nishi, M., Yuhara, A., Obata, A., Fukumoto, S., Hirai, T., Ukita, N., Inoue, T. (1982): JSUM Proceedings, 40, in press.

# ULTRASOUND ESTIMATION OF MYOMETRIAL INVASION OF ENDOMETRIAL CARCINOMA BY USING INTRAUTERINE RADIAL SCANNING

Kaoru Sekiba, Akinori Obata, Nobuo Akamatsu, Nobuaki Ukita and Kuniyasu Niwa

*Department of Obstetrics and Gynecology, Okayama University Medical School, Okayama, Japan*

The prognosis of the endometrial carcinoma is related closely with the degree of histological differentiation(1-2), the degree of myometrial invasion(3-5) and the metastases to lymphnodes(6), and the more undifferentiated carcinoma has the deeper myometrial invasion as well as higher rate of metastasis to regional lymphnodes(3-4). Therefore, it is important to estimate them precisely before treatment. Recently, to the evaluation of myometrial invasion and lymphnode metastasis of the uterine cancer the imaging methods have come to be applied. We have been using ultrasonography(USG)(7-10), X-ray computed tomography(X-ray CT)(8-10) and radioisotope lymphography in this field. In this study, the intrauterine radial scanning, a new technique of USG, has been investigated to estimate the degree of myometrial invasion.

MATERIALS AND METHODS

Twenty cases, who were performed hysterectomies because of emdometrial cancer, were undergone the transabdominal USG and the intrauterine radial scan USG at Okayama University Hospital from January 1980 to December 1981. According to the FIGO staging of endometrial carcinoma, stage Ia were 9 cases, stage Ib 4 cases and stage Ⅱ 7 cases. The transabdominal USG was performed with a full bladder technique by using Aloka SSD 120(2.25 MHz) and SSD 180(3.5 MHz), which are gray scale contact compound scanners, and YEW RT-100(3 MHz) linear electronic scanner. The intrauterine radial scan USG was undergone by inserting a probe of 7 mm in diameter into the uterine cavity (Figure 1). At 1 cm from the tip of the probe a focused concaved transducer of 5 mm in diameter(5 MHz) is attached. The probe was filled with sterilized phisiologic salt solution, and the probe was rotated to perform radial scanning.

The specimen removed by hysterectomy was examined histologically to search the site of the deepest myometrial invasion, and the myometrial invasion was classified into three classes: 1) below one-third(superficial), 2) above one-third but below two-thirds(moderate) and 3) above two-thirds(deep).

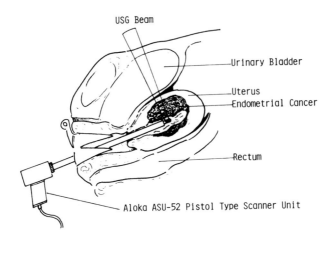

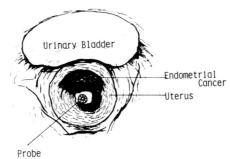

Figure 1. Schema of intrauterine radial scanning

RESULTS

The echo pattern obtained by the transabdominal USG was classified into four types; Type I: anechoic pattern, Type II : linear echo pattern, Type III: cystic echo pattern and Type IV : massive echo pattern, in accordance with the classification of Sekiba and co-workers(7)(Figure 2). The result was that Type I(Figure 3) were observed at four cases(20.0%), Type II (Figure 4) four cases(20.0%), Type III (Figure 5) no case and Type IV (Figure 6) 12 cases(60.0%). By using the echograms obtained by intrauterine radial scanning(Figure 7 and 8). We maesured the thickness of high amplitude irregular shaped solid echo due to carcinoma of the endometrium, and the thickness of the outer part considered as the normal myometrium.

The value of the width of endometrial cancer echo divided by that of carcinoma and normal myometrial echoes was classified into three classes; superficial(below 1/3), moderate(1/3 — 2/3) and deep(above 2/3) invasions.

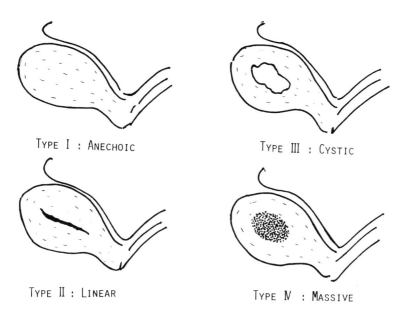

Figure 2. Echographic types of endometrial cancer obtained by transabdominal ultrasonography ( Sekiba, K. et al.(7))

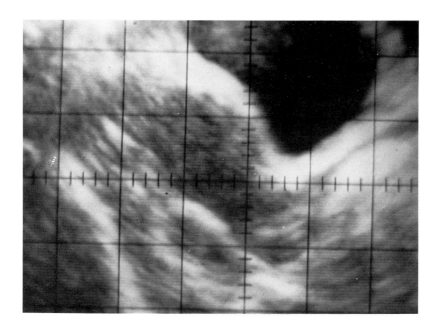

Figure 3. Echogram of Type I —— No abnormal echo is seen interior the uterine body.

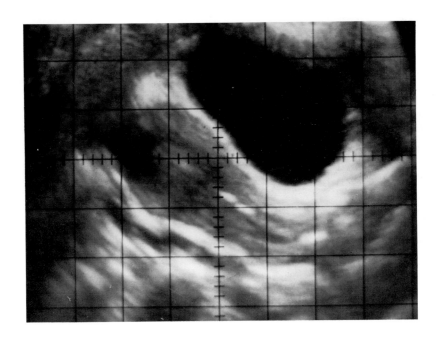

Figure 4. Echogram of Type Ⅱ —— Linear echo is displayed interior the uterus.

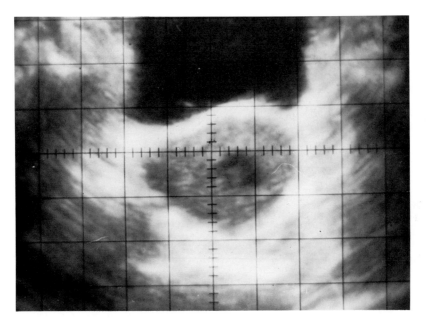

Figure 5. Echogram of Type Ⅲ (transverse section) —— Cystic pattern with surrounding massive echo is visible.

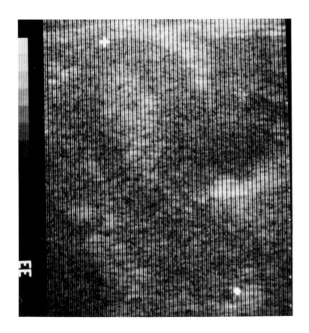

Figure 6 Echogram of Type Ⅳ —— Massive echo with high
amplitude and irregular boundary is seen in the uterus.

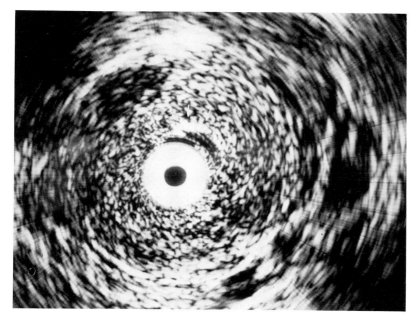

Figure 7. Echogram obtained by intrauterine radial scanning —— case with no myometrial invasion (arrow)

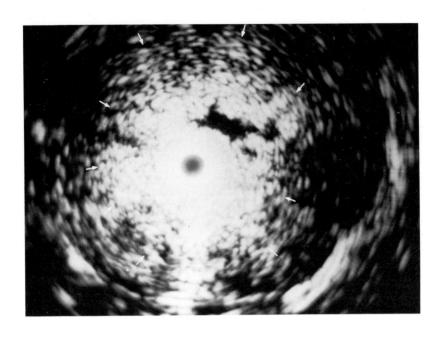

Figure 8. Echogram obtained by intrauterine radial scannig —— case with deep myometrial invasion(arrow).

Five cases were estimated as superficial invasion(—1/3),
9 cases as moderate invasion, and 6 cases as deep invasion. The histological examination of the specimen
revealed 2 cases had superficial myometrial invasion,
9 cases moderate invasion, and 9 cases deep invasion.
    The relation between the type of transabdominal
echo pattern and histological myometrial invasion is
shown in Table 1. All the cases showing Type I and Type
IV had myometrial invasion above 1/3. Type II had 2 cases
of myometrial invasion below 1/3, and 2 cases above 1/3.
The relation between myometrial invasion estimated by
intrauterine radial scanning and that diagnosed histologically is shown in Table 2. In 16 out of 20 cases,
evaluation by radial scan USG and histological evaluation
were in accord, and the correct estimation rate of
intrauterine radial scan USG was 80.0%. In the remaining
4 cases, the radial scan method showed lower estimation
than the histological examination of specimen.

DISCUSSION

    We had performed the transabdominal USG in 59 cases
of endometrial cancer during 8 years from 1973 to 1980,
and the relation between the result of echo pattern
classification and FIGO staging was as in Table 3(11).

Table 1. Correlation between myometrial invasion and transabdominal echographic types

| Type of Echo Pattern | Myometrial Invasion confirmed histologically | | | Total |
|---|---|---|---|---|
| | Superficial ( — 1/3) | Moderate (1/3—2/3) | Deep (2/3— ) | |
| I | 0 | 2 | 2 | 4 |
| II | 2 | 1 | 1 | 4 |
| III | 0 | 0 | 0 | 0 |
| IV | 0 | 6 | 6 | 12 |
| Total | 2 | 9 | 9 | 20 |

Table 2. Correlation between myometrial invasion confirmed histologically and that estimated by intrauterine radial scanning

| Myometrial Invasion estimated by Radial Scan | Myometrial Invasion confirmed histologically | | | Total |
|---|---|---|---|---|
| | Superficial ( — 1/3) | Moderate (1/3— 2/3) | Deep (2/3— ) | |
| Superficial | 2 | 1 | 2 | 5 |
| Moderate | 0 | 8 | 1 | 9 |
| Deep | 0 | 0 | 6 | 6 |
| Total | 2 | 9 | 9 | 20 |

Because all of 20 cases were FIGO stage I and II , the type of echo pattern had a little difference compared with former work. In cases showing Type IV, naturally myometrial invasion was deep. While in Type I the lesion of endometrial cancer was almost small or was not recognized by transabdominal USG. But, 4 cases of Type I had histologically myometrial invasion above 1/3. It seems to show the limit of transabdomenal USG, at least, with the present apparatus.

Therefore, we have tried to use an intrauterine radial scan method. The radial scan method itself has been used in the field of urology to diagnose the prostatic or bladder cancer and evaluate their stages, and the

Table 3. Correlation between FIGO stage and type of transabdominal ultrasonogram

| Type of Echo Pattern | FIGO Stage | | | | | Total |
|---|---|---|---|---|---|---|
| | Ia | Ib | II | III | IV | |
| I | 7 | 2 | 0 | 2 | 2 | 13 |
| II | 5 | 2 | 0 | 0 | 0 | 7 |
| III | 6 | 4 | 2 | 2 | 1 | 15 |
| IV | 10 | 2 | 7 | 1 | 4 | 24 |
| Total | 28 | 10 | 9 | 5 | 7 | 59 |

results have been obtained to show its usefulness(12).

The insertion of transducer into the uterine cavity
can remove the attenuation of ultrasound beam through
the abdominal wall and bladder to the uterine body when
transabdominal USG was undergone. Further, Ultrasound
beam of short wavelength can be used, since the display
field is in short distance. Owing to these advantages,
it can depict well the state of endometrial cancer with
myometrial invasion. As a result, myometrial invasion could be estimated at the correct diagnostic rate as high as
80%, which may be said to show the usefulness of USG with
an intrauterine radial scan method as a new imaging.
However, the present probe has only one fixed transducer,
and can depict a section perpendicular to the axis of
probe. Consequently, the imaging of myometrium in uterine fundus is impossible, and the severe myometrial invasion in this part may be underestimated. At present, the
authers are trying to improve the probe and the transducer to make this weak point better and obtain a conic
section image of uterine fundus.

The development of imaging has been remarkable,
recently, and in addition to supply detailed informations to us. Thus, the authers tried diagnosis of endometrial cancer, the evaluation of myometrial invasion and
lymphnode metastasis with x-ray CT, and obtained fairly
good results. However, the whole body CT requires a
special room and is expensive, while the intrauterine
radial scanner is so simple and inexpensive as to be
used in an internal examination room. So the usefulness
of USG with an intrauterine radial scan method is not
made less valuable. Combining the estimation of
myometrial invasion with an transrectal radial scan method (8,10), the application of USG appears in future to
diagnosis of extent of endometrial carcinoma.

# REFERENCES

1. Cheon, H.(1969): Obstet. Gynecol., 34, 630.
2. Muelenaere, G.F.G.O.(1973): J. Obstet. Gynecol. Br. Commonw., 80, 728.
3. Malkasian, Jr.G.D.(1978): Cancer, 41,996.
4. Kistner, R.W., Kranz, K., Lenherz, T., Lewis, G., Regan, J., Smith, J., Tobin, J., Wied, G.(1973): J. Rep. Med., 10, 53.
5. Homesley, H.D., Boronow, R.C., Lewis, Jr.J.L.(1976): Obstet. Gynecol., 47,100.
6. Morrow, C.P., Di Saia, P.J., Townsend, D.E.(1973): Obstet. Gynecol., Obstet. Gynecol., 42, 399.
7. Sekiba, K., Akamatsu, N., Obata, A., Fukumoto, S., Niwa, K.(1979): IXth FIGO Scientific Exhibition Monograph. p. 36, 213.
8. Sekiba, K., Fujita, T. Akamatsu, N., Obata, A., Fukumoto, S., Goto, R., Hirai, T., Kawai, J., Niwa, K. (1980): JSUM Proceedings, 36, 213.
9. Sekiba, K., Obata, A., Akamatsu, N., Fukumoto, S., Fujita, T., Kawai, J., Hirai, T., Goto, R., Niwa, K. (1980): JSUM Proceedings, 36, 215.
10. Obata, A., Lin, T.T., Fujita, S., Fukumoto, S., Kawai, J., Akamatsu, N., Niwa, K.(1980): Acta Obstet. Gynecol. Jap., 32, 2093.
11. Obata, A.(1981): Acta Obstet. Gynecol. Jap., 33, 2033.
12. Nakamura, S., Niijima, T.(1980): J. Urology, 124, 1980.

# ULTRASONIC EXAMINATION IN GYNECOLOGICAL CANCER

Alfred Kratochwil

*II. Univ. Frauenklinik Wien, Spitalgasse 23, Wien, Austria*

The progress in ultrasonic examination in obstetrics and gynecology within the recent years culminates today in the demand for specific diagnosis of a located tumor. Specifity means however that we are having the macroscopic level and are aiming for histological levels and criterias in our scans. This demand is quite logical but is it realistic as well ? And is it applicable for all genital tumors or only for some of them ?

From the very beginning we have to exclude the uterine lesions such as cervical cancer and to some extent as well the endometrial carcinoma as far as we are concerned with early detection. That means however that we have to concentrate on the tumors of adnexal origin. Compared with the detection of malignancies in great parenchymatous organs such as liver, this goal seems to be much more difficult for tumors of the adnexa.

We are all aware of the high sensitivity of ultrasonic diagnosis of adnexal tumors, but what is to be said about the specifity ? In our daily routine we see quite a lot of gynecological tumors. Although we believe that we have some signs for differentiation between simple cysts, endometriosis and benign teratomas we are always startled about the discrepancies between our assumptions and the histological report. This is quite understandable as the different tumors including as well chronic pelvic inflammatory diseases may have similar echographic appearance.

This is applicable as well for malignant tumors as long as no secondary signs such as complexity of the tumor structure, ascites or liver metastasis and infiltrated omentum make such an assumption probable.

If we are sincere and critical we must confess that our diagnostic conclusions are as well strongly influenced by the patient's history, aspect, the bimanual findings and the laboratory findings.

I dare to doubt that any ultrasonic examiner is able to make a conclusive diagnosis of malignancy without these informations merely evaluating some echographic scans or a videotape where no secondary signs such as ascites etc. exist.

This is not astonishing at all taking into account how
long sometimes a histologist is brooding over a specimen
at his microscope and ordering special stains before
issuing a diagnosis.
This my attitude is only critical and not pessimistic at
all. I believe that it will be possible by the help of
engineers and adaption of computer programs to achieve
a progress in this aforementioned direction as well. I
only want to stress that these at the moment utopic aims
are under research and that we have at the time no possibility for early detection of an ovarian carcinoma.

But nevertheless there exists a wide field of application of ultrasonic examination techniques for preoperative outlining of the tumor, in radio therapy-planning
and in the follow-up of tumors after irradiation and
chemotherapy to control the therapeutic effect and to lo-
cate local and lymphonodal recurrences after radical
surgery.

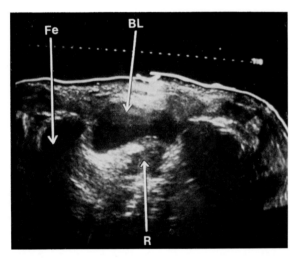

Fig. 1. Recurrence of a Wertheim's operation. Transverse
scan. Fe = femural head, Bl = bladder, R = recurrence.


After these critical introductorial remarks let us have
a look for the benefits of ultrasonic diagnosis in gynecological cancers. As it already was pointed out that
tumor growth in the uterus can only be detected in far advanced stages when the tumor has outgrown the organ´s
border. In case of a cervical cancer,this is the case if
the tumor grows towards the rectum or has infiltrated the
bladder (Fig. 1 ). In these cases the infiltrating process within the bladder can be outlined.
This is similar as well for endometrial carcinomas. So
f.i. when in an old aged woman beyond the menopause a lar-

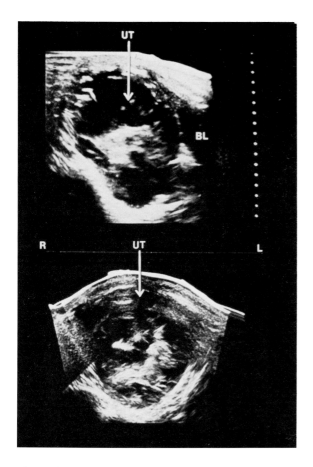

Fig. 2. Far advanced endometrial carcinoma. Upper scan: longitudinal scan in the midline. UT = uterus, BL = bladder. Lower scan: transverse scan.

ge thin-walled uterus containing solid and cystic parts can be outlined (Fig. 2), or the tumor-growth has penetrated the uterine wall.

An ovarian cancer may be suspected if the tumor demonstrates a relatively complex structure with big irregular solid masses (Fig. 3), or thickened septs in which broad solid masses can be outlined.
The assumption of malignancy becomes certainity if ascites can be detected. This ascites must not necessarily be anechoic but may contain as well weak echoes as in haemorrhagic or chyloic ascites.

According to the peritoneal metastasis the bowel in these cases is not free to float on the fluid as it would be expected due to its gaseous content. The loops are fixed and retracted towards the mesenteric root.
In cases of ovarian cancer it is mandatory as well to

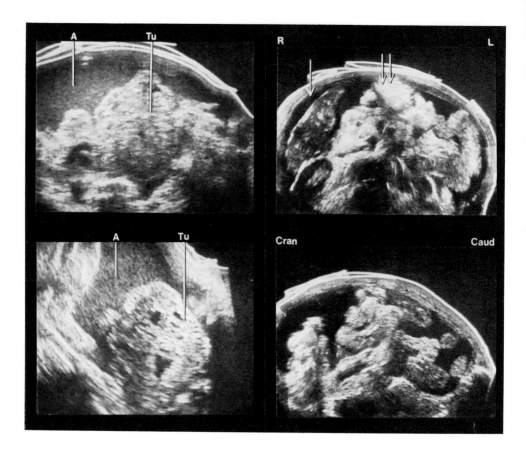

Fig. 3. Ovarian cancer with haemorrhagic ascites, upper scan: transverse scan, below: longitudinal scan. Tu = tumour, A = ascites, containing fine echoes due to haemorrhagic ascites.

Fig. 4. Malignant ascites, liver metastasis and omental infiltration (double arrow).

examine the upper abdomen to inspect the liver for secondaries (Fig. 4) and to look for an infiltrated omentum which presents as a thickened parallel structure beneath the abdominal wall.Of special interest in this connection is the careful observation of the right hemidiaphragm in search for tumor-seeds which can be detected from a dimension of 1 cm onwards. Smaller lesions will escape the ultrasonic evaluation.
The experienced ultrasonic examiner may sometimes make for the referring clinician a surprising diagnosis in cases of suspected ovarian lesions. If a clinical suspected ovarian tumor proofs at ultrasonic examination to be irregular and somewhat polycyclic and broadly attached to the pelvic wall, the upper abdomen has to be inspected

immediately. In such cases not only an enlarged liver and spleen may be found, but as well polycyclic areas in front of the spine along the aorta reaching to the liver hilum so that immediately a systemic disease as Hodgkin´s disease may be assumed. Similar pictures may be produced as well by retroperitoneal metastasis of melanoma and in sarcoma originated from the fatty tissue.

In cases of ovarian cancers referred for a second-look-operation ultrasonic examination may be useful to outline ascites and the amount of the rest tumor after a prior operation.

In comparison with CT scanning, the CT is sometimes better in outlining the extent of the tumor towards the neighbouring organs such as rectosigmoid and bladder.

Echography has as well its place in radiotherapy-treatment planning if no CT is available. By ultrasonic examination the patient´s body contour can be clearly outlined and the tumor as well. The distance from the anterior and the posterior surface and the tumor volume can be exactly estimated. By an interface it is possible to link the ultrasonic machine with the computer to fit the isodoses and the ports of irradiation individually as long as the patient is in therapy position.

The tumor measurements form as well the basis for therapy control. Several ultrasonic measurements during the course of the treatment demonstrate clearly if the tumor is responding or not.

Echography is as well of advantage in the detection of local or lymphonodal recurrences after radical treatment of gynecological cancer. Echography is in these cases superior to lymphangio- and scintigraphy, because these methods are bound to a functioning lymphatic system,which is however distroyed by the radical treatment.

Echography is able however to outline the lesions. Of course, this method is not able to detect early lesions as the lesions must measure at least 2 cm before they become demonstrable. In these cases the upper abdomen has to be inspected as well as to exclude or proof hydrone-phrosis caused by ureteral obstruction. In this connection it should be mentioned as well that ultrasonic exa-mination of the kidneys is favourable as well after radi-cal surgery to minimize radiation, or where i.v.P. is otherwise impossible or contraindicated.

Ultrasonic examination after surgery can be applied suc-cessfully to detect the causes of unexplained fever and pains. These symptoms might be caused by haematomas, abs-cesses or lymphcysts which might be mimicking as well an an early recurrence.

I hope that I could point out the manifold possibilities of ultrasonic examinations in conjunction with gynecolo-gical cancers. Although we are at the time unable to make a conclusive diagnosis of malignancy only based on ultra-sonid examinations, the efforts in this direction should be multiplied but critically controlled.

# DIAGNOSTIC APPLICATIONS OF ULTRASOUND IN UTERINE TUMORS

G. Maresca, P. Mirk, A.M. De Gaetano, S. Speca and C. Colagrande

*Istituto di Radiologia, Università Cattolica S. Cuore, Rome, Italy*

The ultrasonographic findings in 30 patients affected by uterine tumors (adenocarcinoma of the cervix, endometrial carcinoma, sarcoma, choriocarcinoma) are described. Out of the 30 patients, 13 had not received any previous treatment; 17 had already been treated with surgery or radiotherapy and were evaluated for suspected recurrence. In the authors' experience US examination (always to be performed after clinical evaluation) is not suitable for diagnosing the disease, but it may prove helpful in preoperative assessment since it can demonstrate the local extent of the tumor at the vaginal cuff and into the parametria, as well as a possible involvement of the ureters and the bladder. Enlarged lymph nodes may be detected but are more reliably assessed by CT; invasion of the rectum is even more difficult to assess and usually may only be suggested by US alone. It is also possible to evaluate by US the response to radiation and perfusional endoarterial chemotherapy, not only when gynecological examination is difficult (fibrosis, scarrings, local tenderness) but especially so in all emergency situations that such treatments may cause.

# OVARIAN TUMORS: POSSIBLE ULTRASONIC DISTINCTION BETWEEN BENIGN AND MALIGNANT?

Salvator Levi, Joëlle Awoust and Anne Carton

*Ultrasound Laboratory, Department of Gynecology and Obstetrics, University Hospital Brugmann, 1020 Brussels, Belgium*

The discovery of ovarian tumors is frequent in gynecological practice. Ovarian pathology gathers a great variety of abnormalities: from hyperplasy till tumors measuring about forthy centimeters and weighing several pounds.

Ultrasonography enables to obtain images of the ovaries whatever their size may be and even shows the aspects of their physiological changes during the menstrual cycle: growth, maturation and rupture of follicles and their transformation in corpus luteum (Fig.1). Consequently, any morphological change of the ovary is descriptible.

The first ovarian tumor displayed by ultrasound was described by Donald in 1958 (1). Techniques have been improved since then and ultrasonography is now an important tool for the diagnosis of pelvic diseases and especially ovarian tumors.

According to the authors, the ratio of correct results varies from 80 to 95 % (2-7). Moreover, for some of them, the difference between benign and malignant tumors can be assessed with ultrasonography (6-10). We suggest the reader to examine the echographic signs which might help to characterize benign or malignant tumors.

Ultrasonograms of pelvic tumors can show a highly variety of images: size, shape, echo-signals distribution and surrounding changes are very different indeed. Tumors are presumed to be of ovarian origin considering their **position** compared to the noticeable vicinal structures: uterus, vagina, pelvic walls, bladder, Douglas pouch (Fig.1); more exceptionnal and for small tumors only, by the **connection** with their vessels or infundibulo-pelvic ligaments.

## THE LOCALIZATION

Tumor localization varies mainly according to the size of the tumor: in the pelvis and lateral to the uterus when its size is under 5-6 cm (Fig.1), rather deep in the pelvis and behind the uterus in the Douglas pouch when its size is somewhat larger (Fig.2 A,B,D,E). Tumors lie beyond the uterus and above the pelvis brim, on the whole or partly, when it is still larger (Fig.2 A,C,F); excepted in cases where adherencies keep the tumor in the pelvis. No matter the localization might be, it is not a criteria enabling to determine benignity or malignity. Adherencies sticking some tumors in the pelvis may go with both benign (endometriosis) and malignant tumors (invading the vicinal structures).

## THE SIZE

The size of ovarian tumors can be very different. Ovarian diameters vary from single to double in physiological conditions, related to age, parity and even the menstrual cycle. The growth of the graafian follicle on one or both sides alters the size, depending on the amount and degree of follicle development. The menstrual variation of small cystic tumor is a good omen of benignity. The visualization of many micro-cystic structures (from 2 to 10 mm), varying little and often present in both ovaries, are not alarming; they are often related to functionnal disturbances (Fig.1 D-G). Apart from the above mentionned cases, the abnormalities of size are to be considered at first as a tumor. Tumors may both be benign or malignant no matter their volume (4 to 40 cm) according to the stage at the observation time. They all start their evolution at a normal size.

## THE SHAPE

Organ or tumor shapes depend mainly on both its size and contents (fluid, solid) and secondly on the environment. Normal size and hypertrophic ovary (Fig.1 A,C,D) display an oval shape in the two scans section, parasagittal and transverse. Beyond that, the oval image tends to become circle shape image displayed in the two perpendicular sections; it corresponds to a spheric tumor (Fig.1,E;Fig.3 C,D). If the diameters still increase,the shape becomes oval again, the environment producing progressive deformations (Fig.2D,F;Fig.3A,B;Fig.4). Nevertheless, the contents may alter the typical changes in shape evolution: an almost solid tumor escapes this rule, it keeps nearly spherical shape and the contours are less regular, somewhat dented (Fig.5). The tumor limit, at the opposite side of the transducer, is sometimes not well visualized, that sign being due to the content of the tumor which strongly absorbes the sound energy. Rather alarming, it corresponds often to a carcinoma but also to a Brenner tumor (seldom malignant) or to an ovarian fibroma. The shape also fails to indicate a tendency to benignity or malignancy.

## THE INTERNAL ASPECT

Internal aspect of the tumor corresponds to the presence (or absence), within the tumor walls, of echoes and echo-distribution, amplitude of echo-signals, etc.
The images will be classified into three groups: 1. **tumors mainly non-echogenic**; 2. **tumors mainly echogenic** and 3. **mixed tumors**, with echoic- and anechoic areas.

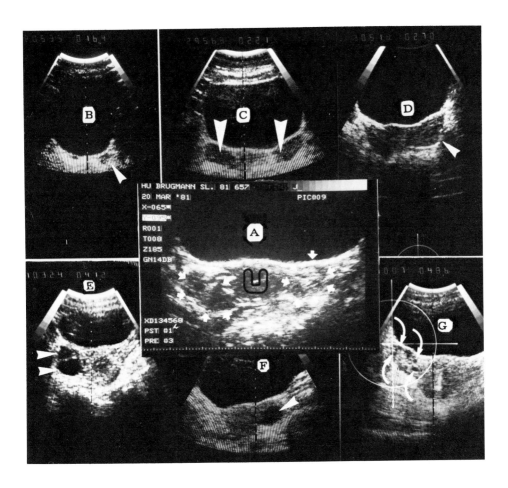

*Figure* 1. NORMAL ASPECT AND SMALL CHANGES IN THE OVARIES
(transverse scans).
A. Normal size and normal echogeneicity of both ovaries
(showed by arrows); between the ovaries, the corpus uteri
(u); above these structures, the black area corresponds
to the full bladder.
B. Hypotrophic ovaries in 11 years-old girl : left ovary
shown by arrow.
C. Normal size ovaries (28yr, II para).
D. Hypertrophic ovary (arrow).
E. Small follicular cysts (two arrows); cysts edges are
more sharp than the follicles shown in F.
F. Ovarian mature follicle (23 X 19 mm, arrow).
G. Micropolycystic right ovary (on the left); very small
cysts are well visible, some of them are shown by arrows;
detection is less due to the anechoic area than the posterior enhancement;the larger cyst has a 4 mm diameter.

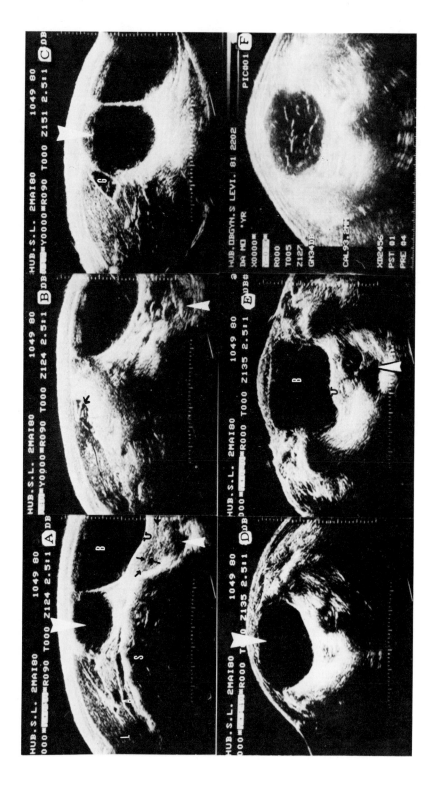

*Figure 2*

*Figure* 2. A-E : Pelvis and abdomen containing two different tumors: an UNILOCULAR SEROUS CYSTADENOMA and a PSEUDOMUCINOUS CYSTADENOMA (small arrow).
A. Sagittal section : bladder (B), uterus (U), uterine cavity (black arrows), pseudomucinous cyst in the Douglas pouch on the right (small white arrow), serous cyst is high in the abdomen and on the left (big white arrow), liver (L), aorta (A), spine (S)(scale2.5:1).
B. Left parasagittal section (4cm from midline), bladder, duodenum (black arrow), multilocular pseudomucinous cyst.
C. Parasagittal section, 4 cm right to the median line, serous cyst, galbladder (G).
D. Transverse horizontal section, 14 cm above symphysis pubis,serous cyst with posterior enhancement.
E. Transverse horizontal section, 2 cm above symphysis pubis,showing to the right a pseudomucinous cyst, bladder, uterus.
F. Transverse section of another case : serous cyst with many echoes inside, simulating a multilocular cyst; macroscopic examination of the tumor showed a unilocular cyst containing fibrin deposits.

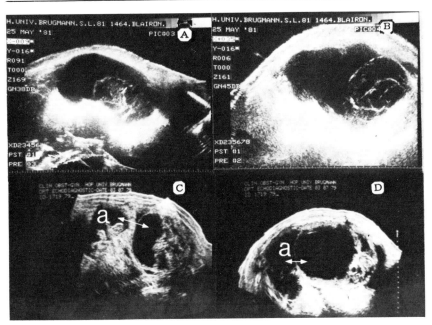

*Figure* 3. A-B : BENIGN PSEUDOMUCINOUS CYST of the left ovary,dimensions at laparotomy were 23 x 17 x 11 cm and it weight was 2.5kg; a smooth enveloppe-containing numerous small cysts at the lower part of the tumor, to the right side. The contours are rather irregular. No ascitis. C-D : PSEUDOMUCINOUS MALIGNANT CYST of the left ovary, weighing 2.0kg and 17 cm diameter in size. C.:To the right, numerous echoes and a free-echo area forms the tumor; to the left, ascitis(a) with floating bowels. The wall in between is thick (arrow).
D.:The tumor is on the right and ascitis (a) on the left; the wall between the tumor and ascitis zone is very thin (arrow). Both tumors AB and CD were suspected of malignancy.

## 1. Tumors mainly non-echogenic

Non-echogenic means that within the reflective envelope, a non-reflective material can be found. Even the visualization of small dots within the tumor has no really significance: they are not echoes reflected by elements, but are the result of a scatter phenomenon.

A totaly echofree area suggests a perfect homogeneity of the medium (ex.bladder,Fig.2 E). Only liquid tumors, without any solid element such as cells, fibrin, cristals, show this characteristic; echofree tumors are met in some unilocular serous cystadenomas (Fig.2 A,C,D). Moreover, if the image of the envelope is very regular, smooth inside and outside, what indicates a probable absence of vegetations, the tumor may be classified among the benign ones (Fig.2 D). The papillary vegetations can indeed be revealed, according to their size, either by reflection or scattering of sound energy. The low attenuation of ultrasound in liquid, added to the change in sound- velocity between tissues and liquids, increase the reflection on the posterior wall of the tumor and even deeper (Fig.2 C).

Frequently, cystic liquid areas are crossed by walls which form unequal sized compartiments: the dividing membranes produce typical reflections, some are thin, some others thick (Fig.4). The amount, surface and volume of the chambers are determined by several scans made at regular and short intervals. The size and number of cystic-chambers are variable.It concerns multilocular cystic tumors: serous- and pseudomucinous-cystadenomas (Fig.3 A,B). Their surface is often irregular, due to nodules of tissue, pediculated or not. On the inside of cystic walls, vegetations are more visible than on the outside because they are better defined when surrounded by serous or mucinous liquid. These tumors may be either benign or malignant, in particular if the tumor is serous, which is very difficult indeed to determine as to refute. The macroscopic aspect of the tumor does not enable to make the difference; only microscopy can do so. However, the mucinous matter sometimes produces a very low scattering and very weak signals. If it is possible to assess that the matter is mucinous, then the risk of malignancy is not higher than 5 % (Fig.2 B,D,E;Fig.3 C,D).

## 2. Tumors mainly echogenic

The inside of the envelope, or capsule, which is - as for the cysts - displayed because the difference of impedances between vicinal tissues, is filled with solid tissue.

Homogeneous or not, very dense or not, the tissue is more or less well irrigated by blood.

Different echographic pictures correspond to those different structural characteristics. A very homogeneous tumor provides few echoes and of generally low amplitude;they are due to the variable distribution of tissue layers and vessels crossed by sound waves. The tumor echoes increased in amount and amplitude with the tissue heterogeneicity. The density of the tumoral tissue - loose or tight, oedematous

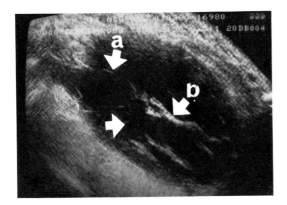

*Figure* 4. BENIGN SEROUS
CYSTADENOMA, this is an
example where thin(a) and
thick(b) walls delineating
compartiments can be found
in the same benign tumor.

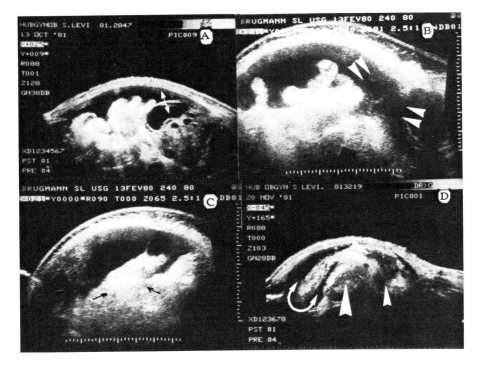

*Figure* 5. SOLID TUMORS.
A. SOLID MALIGNANT TUMOR containing sonolucent areas due to necrosis
(one arrow) and hemorrage (two arrows).
B. BENIGN LUTEOMA : the walls are well defined, the inside of the
tumor is like as *Figure* A.
C.and D. SOLID MALIGNANT TUMOR on the left (big arrow) and BENIGN
OVARIAN HYPERPLASIA, on the right (small arrow). The left measures:
85 x 50 x 60 mm, the right : 50 x 40 x 30 mm, both ovaries have the
same appearance and the same unclear-defined contours.

or dried up - is partly responsible for the absorption of sound energy. The absorption alters the visibility of the deepest edge of tumor (Fig.5).

The irrigation - arterial, venous and lymphatic - can be normal, excessive or inadequate. Irrigation plays an important role in imaging because it modify greatly the macroscopic and echographic aspects of the tumor. When vascularity is rich, it provides many sources of reflections. If it is weak, the tumor becomes necrotic and produces very echogenic areas (Fig.5). With poor draining, oedema appears and sonar transmission and reflection increase. Blood vessels inside the tumor are eventually dammaged by the tumoral process: a local hemorrage happens and changes the echo-distribution.Mineral deposit, mainly calcium, comes from an altered irrigation and may produce strong echoes. These echo densities are sometimes accompanied by shadowing, according to the use of single or compound scans. Shadowing can either be due to the reflection or to important absorption.If they are very small, calcifications produce only scattering.

Echogenic tumors are thus displayed by very different patterns and are therefore seldom characteristic of one of tumor. They will be called ovarian carcinoma whatever their precise origin may be: papillary serous and pseudomucinous cystadenoma, endometrioid, non-differentiated. They might be also mesonephroma, dysgerminoma which are also malignant. The same aspect may also correspond to a tumor of low potential of malignity (10 to 30 %): granulosa cell tumor, arrhenoblastoma (10 % of the echogenic tumors). Benign tumors give sometimes complex pictures: fibroma, fibro-adenoma; their potential of malignancy is extremely low.

3. **Mixed tumors or partly echogenic and partly non-echogenic**

Except the echogenic tumors with only minor tissue alterations producing some small non-echogenic areas, the difference between mainly echogenic and mixed tumors seems to be artificial. Though it enables to classify the tumors which contain reflecting and non reflecting areas from their origin, counter to many echogenic tumors where sonolucent areas appear later on in their evolution (Fig.6 A,B).

This group includes mainly teratomas. They are frequent (about 15% out of ovarian tumors) but seldom malignant (about 2 %).

Macroscopically very polymorph,they display thus a variety of echographic pictures, according to the variety of possible components including cysts filled with hair, serous- spumous- or oily- material, bone, teeth or cartilage. The areas of dense tissue may correspond to a malignant transformation. As well as in the former described tumors, necrotic or suppurating areas can be observed.

In the best cases, the most typical areas are poorly    echoic with some strong reflections and shadows which make the diagnosis easier. Donald (11) emphazised the difficulty of the right diagnosis of ovarian teratomas and all the authors agree with his conclusions. Because this

172

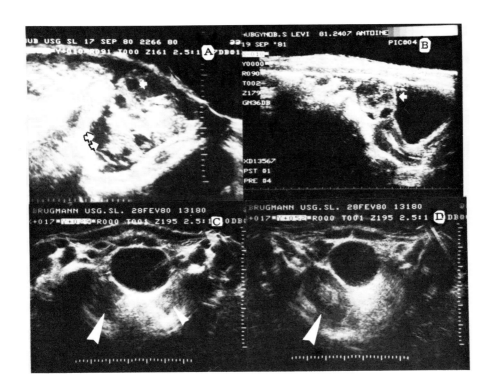

*Figure* 6. ASCITIS AND CARCINOMATOSIS PERITONEALIS.
A. HYBRID PELVIC TUMOR; on this longitudinal scan, the tumor is
well delimited on the right from the ascitis (arrows) in which
the bowels are floating.
B. ENDOMETRIOID CARCINOMA (6 cm diameter) with ascitis and free·
floating bowels; the tumor is on the right and very bad delineated
on this longitudinal scan (arrows).
C. ENDOMETRIOID CARCINOMA : on this image, bowels are fixed to the
meso (arrows).
D. SOLID OVARIAN CARCINOMA : ascitis fluid is divided (thin arrows)
by septa due to peritoneal carcinomatosis, bowels (small arrow)
are sticky on the solid tumor (big arrow).

tumor is either solid (25%), either cystic (25%) and most often mixed (we classified it in this last group), the correct diagnosis is only obtained in about half of the cases (3,12). Here again a high polymorphism of the sonograms is responsible of many false diagnoses: true cancers diagnosed as teratomas and vice-versa (12).

## THE ENVIRONMENT OF THE TUMOR - THE METASTASES - THE BILATERALITY

The outline has to be distinguished from the shape of the tumor. The shape is proper to it but outline depends on the structure of the capsule and on the reaction of the vicinal structures. A tumor may be round and smooth, with buds on the outside, covered in whole or partially by vegetations, closely adherent to the surrounding tissue or invading them. The papillar extracystic proliferation of multilocular serous tumors can be observed as well on benign tumors as in malignant ones. Microscopy only enables the distinction. Unilocular serous cysts of middle size have sometimes proliferations even they are often benignant. Exophytic vegetations of pseudo-mucinous tumors neither are a wittness of malignity.

In 20 to 25 % of the cases, malignant arrhenoblastoma **do not** adhere to the vicinal tissue; but if tumor is adherent, **it is** a sign of malignity in case of granulosa tumors as well in mesonephroma.

External vegetations are displayed as an irregular outline with small very reflective areas. Imprecise outline, without clear difference between the tumor and vicinal structures, may be the signs of adherences. Then, the tumor appears to be greater than it is really. The reactions between the tumor and vicinal structures can go beyond the stage of inflammatory process and adherences. Invasion is a sign of malignity to be searched (Fig.6 D).

The invasion is suspected if the limit of a part of the tumor is not clearly defined. But peri-tumoral inflammatory processes show the same defects on the outlines (Fig.6 B). The rupture of the tumor is often a sign of malignity: the outline is no longer visible, the liquid included in the cyst sheds in the abdominal cavity.

The rupture of mucinous cysts is followed by an invasion of the peritoneal cavity and formation of granuloma; risk of malignity is higher then (pseudomyxoma).

Cyst rupture is not clearly identified on pictures and the reasons misunderstanding are many: the liquid shed from the cyst does not differ so much from ascitis,the peritoneum from the enveloppe of the tumor and compartimented ascitis from damaged cystic part (Fig.6 D).

Other reactions, like ascitis, are easy to demonstrate by echography.

Ascitis accompanies often malignant tumor such as ovarian solid-carcinoma, mesonephroma, dysgerminoma, malignant tumors of the granulosa cells. Though ascitis is also a complication of one third out of the ovarian fibroma (with or without hydrothorax in Demons-Meigs' syndroma) and of benign tumors

174

of the granulosa. Ascitis, especially when it is abundant in abdomen and pelvis, helps to the echographic observation of peritoneal extension, an other sign of malignity. Pathologists emphazise often on the fact that some cancerous cysts can not be clearly defined even microscopically in certain tumors with ascitis and peritoneum nodules.

Signs at some distance of the tumor may add to malignity risks: hypertrophic lymph nodes (pelvic and para-aortic), and liver metastases. The detection of these signs help certainly to the diagnosis of malignity but somewhat late (6,8-11).

Bilaterality of a tumor is a presumption of malignity. Except the cases when the tumor is much greater than the other pelvic organs, it should be possible to detect and describe the second ovary.

How will help the observation of ovarian enlargment on the other side ? The observation of abnormalities to assess the risk of malignity ? Once again, bilaterality is a variable sign which is not significant: serous cystadenocarcinoma are bilateral in about half of the cases, benign cysts in one out off five cases. Mucinous malignant tumors are bilateral in about one out four cases against one out ten if they are benign. Solid carcinoma (mainly echogenic) are bilateral only one out five case and fibroma one out ten. The other benign and malignant tumors have variable proportions in their bilateral characteristic.

## CONCLUSIONS

The ultrasonographic image of the ovarian cancer is not more significant than the macroscopic one. Ultrasonographic examination can only suggest presumptions which can help for diagnostic added to other signs.All of them together can reinforced the statistical risk of malignancy. Sekiba calculated the risk of malignancy with a serie of criterias as explained in the following chapter. For a long time, Donald (11) and Kratochwil (13) described the presumptive signs of malignancy: the more complicated the picture is, the higher the risk of malignancy is. More precise criteria help considerably to quantify and assess the risk: echogenic or mixed tumor (3-5,9-11),irregular outline (7-10), multilocular structure (6-10,14), thickness of septa (6,7,9), great size (3,4,6-8). The coexisting signs increase the presumptions which are mainly absolute when they concern epiploon metastasis (10,11,14), lymph nodes enlargement (9,10) or liver metastasis (9-11), a little less for ascitis (7-11).

If it is true that the majority of observed abnormalities are neither specific of malignity or benignity, ultrasonography enables to detect, describe, measure and eventually follow the evelution of the tumor and lesions after chemical and radiation treatment.When the outlines are not clearly visualized , CT-Scan achieved the examination by demonstration the integrity of the capsule or the invasion of the vicinal structures.

# REFERENCES

1. **DONALD I., McVICAR J., BROWN T.G.:** "Investigation of abdominal masses by pulsed ultrasound". Lancet 1: 1188-1194, 1958.
2. **LEVI S.:** "Le diagnostic des tumeurs gynécologiques" Schw.Gynaek.und Geburts. 2: 11-24, 1971.
3. **COCHRANE W.J., THOMAS M.A.:** "Ultrasound diagnosis of gynecologic pelvic masses". Radiology 110: 649-654, 1974.
4. **LEVI S., DELVAL R.:** "Value of ultrasonic diagnosis of gynecological tumours in 370 surgical cases". Act.Obs.Gyn.Scand. 55: 261-266, 1976.
5. **QUINONES C.Y.** in "Ultrasonic examination in gynecology" In A.Kratochwil : Progress in Medical Ultrasound, volume 2 (ed.A.Kurjak), Excerpta Medica, Amsterdam 1981, p.105-110.
6. **MEIRE H.B., FARRANT P., GUHA T.:** "Distinction of benign from malignant ovarian cysts by ultrasound". Br.J.Obs.Gyn. 85: 893-899, 1978.
7. **SEKIBA K., FUKUMOTO S., FUJITA T., AKAMATSU N.:** "Computer assisted ultrasound diagnosis of ovarian tumor". In:Recent Advances in Ultrasound Diagnosis 3 (ed.A.Kurjak and A.Kratochwil), Excerpta Medica, Amsterdam, 1981, p.295-299.
8. **KOBAYASHI M.:** "Use of diagnostic ultrasound in trophoblastic neoplasms and ovarian tumors". Cancer: 441-452, 1976.
9. **WALSH J.W., TAYLOR K.J., WASSON J.F.** : "Gray scale ultrasound in 204 proved gynecologic masses: accuracy and specific diagnostic criteria" Radiology 130: 391-397, 1979.
10.**KRATOCHWIL A.:** "Ultrasonic examination in gynecological tumors". In: Recent Advances in Ultrasound Diagnosis 3 (ed.A.Kurjak and A.Kratochwil), Excerpta Medica, Amsterdam, 1981, p.284-289.
11.**DONALD I.:** "Ultrasound in the diagnosis of ovarian neoplasia". In:Diagnosis and treatment of ovarian neoplasic alterations", Excerpta Medica ICS 364, Amsterdam, 1974, p.92-98.
12.**FUKUMOTO S., SEKIBA K., FUJITA T. et al.:** "Gray scale ultrasound imaging of the benign ovarian teratoma". Excerpta Medica ICS 547, Amsterdam, 1981, p.51.
13.**KRATOCHWIL A.:** "Sonography in Gynaecology" In:Present and Future of Diagnostic Ultrasound (ed.I.Donald and S.Levi), Kooyker Scient.Public., Rotterdam, 1976, p.63-75.
14.**QUEENAN J.T., KUBARYCH S.F., DOUGLAS D.L.:** "Evaluation of diagnostic ultrasound in gynecology". Am.J.Obs.Gyn.123: 453-465, 1975.
15.**GOMPEL C., SILVERBERG S.:** "Pathology in gynecology and obstetrics", Presses Académiques Européennes, Brussels, 1969.

# VALIDITY OF ULTRASOUND DIAGNOSIS OF OVARIAN CARCINOMA

F. Destro, P.L. Ceccarello, F. Calcagnile, M. Lando, E. Meli and M. Destro

*Department of Obstetrics and Gynecology, City Hospital of Gorizia, Gorizia, Italy*

## INTRODUCTION

The present growing interest in Ultrasound diagnosis springs from the fact that it can be of great help in giving the most correct diagnosis possible when there is a lack or absence of objective clinical data. In fact, as far as Obstetrics is concerned this methodology represents a part of semeiotics which is, at present, irreplaceable. Can the same be said with regards to Gynaecology?

## PURPOSE OF THE INVESTIGATION

The aim of this investigation is that of assessing the significance of ultrasound diagnosis in Gynaecology and in what way it can help the clinician to obtain the most correct diagnosis possible.

This investigation considers only the soundness and significance of ultrasound diagnosis as far as malignant solid and cystic tumors of the ovary are concerned.

## MATERIAL AND METHOD

To carry out our research we took into consideration, only and exclusively, those random cases in which the clinical and ecographical examinations were made independently, one from the other, and the results obtained were in their turn compared with the anatomical and histopathological ones.

As a result of our criterion in selecting cases, the survey was limited to only 27 cases which came under our observation from January 1st 1972 to June 15th 1981.

The ecographic examination was carried out by means of the following equipment:
1)    Kretz Technik 4100 MGS
      from 1970 to 1976

2)   Picker – Echoview system 8OL – 8OC
     from 1976 up to and including today
3)   Superscan 50
     from April 1980 up to and including today.
Of the three types of equipment used, those which gave the most detailed data, because they were supplied with the grey scale, were those given by No. 2 and No. 3.

In order to obtain the most correct diagnosis possible we made use, during the investigation and afterwards, of standards already stated by Ianniruberto et al. (2), by Meire et al. (3), and by Takeuchi et al. (5).

## SURVEY

Cases of malignant solid and cystic neoplasy of the ovary with their respective significance in comparison with clinical and histopathological diagnosis are reported in Tables 1 and 2.

## COMMENT AND RESULTS

From the data that emerge from our survey of random cases there is no significance if we compare the ecographical report with the clinical one.

It is in fact well known that the present technical possibilities innate in ultrasonography are not yet able to give a characterization of the tissues examined.

In order to obtain such a result it would be necessary to put into clinical practice the proposals suggested by Herment (1) and by Nicholas (4). In fact the former suggests the study and differentiation of the various tissues by means of "impediography" the latter by means of "diffraction".

To sum up, taking for granted the fact that the technical and clinical preparation of the person carrying out the ultrasound investigation, it must be maintained that, at the present level of knowledge and remembering the technical possibilities of the equipment usually used, ultrasound investigation cannot be considered as a determinant in the sphere of gynaecological diagnosis, and in this specific case, in the diagnosis of malignant neoplasy of the ovary. It is thus to be considered, despite misleading appearances, a complementary examination.

178

TABLE 1.    Malignant cystic neoformations

Number of cases for anatomical histopathological report: No. 12

Correspondence of clinical diagnosis in 4 cases (33,33 %)

Correspondence of ecographic diagnosis in 8 cases (66,67 %)

Significance of ecographic diagnosis compared with the clinical one

$$x^2 = 2,68 \qquad p > 0,05$$

TABLE 2.    Malignant solid neoformations (ovarian)

Number of cases for anatomical histopathological report: No. 15

Correspondence of clinical diagnosis in 9 cases (60 %)

Correspondence of ecographic diagnosis in 10 cases (66,66 %)

Significance of ecographic diagnosis compared with the clinical one

$$x^2 = 0,13 \qquad p > 0,7$$

179

REFERENCES

1. Herment,A. (1980): "Impediography"; principle, applicability, results. In: Thijssen, J.M. (Rd): Ultrasonic tissue characterization clinical achievements and technological potentials. Stafleu's Scientific Publishing Company. Alphen aan den Rijn/Brussels, The Netherlands.
2. Ianniruberto,A., Destro,F. and Ceccarello,P.L. (1974): Il Sonar in Ostetricia e Ginecologia. Verduci Edizioni Scientifiche, Roma.
3. Meire,H.B., Farrant,P. and Guha,T. (1978): Distinction of benign from malignant ovarian cysts by ultrasound. Br. J. Obstet. Gynaecol. 85,893.
4. Nicholas,D. (1980): Interference effects in the Backscattered signals from Human tumors. In: Thijssen,J.M. (Ed): Ultrasonic tissue characterization clinical achievements and technological potentials. Stafleu's Scientific Publishing Company. Alphen aan den Rijn/Brussels, The Netherlands.
5. Takeuchi,H., Kawamata,C., Sugie,T. and Kobayashi,T. (1978): Gray-scale ultrasonic diagnosis of ovarian carcinoma. In: Kurjak,A. (Ed.): Recent advances in Ultrasound. Vol. I, Excerpta Medica, Amsterdam, The Netherlands., pp.113.

# COMPUTER ASSISTED ULTRASOUND DIAGNOSIS OF OVARIAN MALIGNANCY

Kaoru Sekiba, Nobuo Akamatsu, Satoru Fukumoto, Takuo Fujita, Takeshi Hirai[1] and Nobutaka Tsubota[2]

[1]*Department of Obstetrics and Gynecology, Okayama University Medical School, Okayama and* [2]*Department of Hygiene, Hiroshima University Medical School, Hiroshima, Japan*

Cervical cancer, which occurs the highest frequency of malignant tumor in gynecologic field, can usually be detected at an early stage and healed frequently, because symptoms such as irregular vaginal bleeding often occur, vaginoscopical and colposcopical observations can easily be done, and further a punch biopsy can be conducted. In the case of ovarian malignancy, however, no symptoms can be observed at an early stage. It is difficult to determine whether a slightly enlarged ovary is benign or malignant only by bimanual examination. Thus most ovarian cancer had been able to identify only after laparotomy.

The ultrasonography(USG), as a diagnostic method by imaging, has found extensive application because the apparatus is smallsized and very handy. The USG, which was efficient for discrimination between cystic mass and solid mass, has been used for diagnosis of ovarian tumor and uterine myoma as well. Recently, the improved USG system has made it possible to discribe the difference in the delicate structure interior the mass, so that it can be applied for discrimination between benign and malignant tumor.

The former method of reading the USG images, though it was an objective observation method, largely depend on the observers, sensitivity, technical skill and experience, thus resulting in greatly varying diagnoses. In 1977 Takeuch and his coworkers (1) analyzed the echograms of 500 ovarian tumors to establish a diagnostic standard for judging the degree of malignancy of an ovarian tumor. Since then procedures with better objectivity, including our method, for diagnosing ovarian malignancy and judging degree of malignancy, have been devised(2-5).

We have independently conducted computed analysis of the echo patterns on ovarian tumor by the use of gray scale untrasound. We have also reviewed a weighted scoring system to judge the degree of malignancy of ovarian tumor. Recently, its prospective application has been performed.

## ANALYSIS OF ECHO PATTERNS

During the period of 5 years from January 1975 to

Table 1 Number of tumors at each histological classifica-tion

| Histological Group | | No. of Tumor | |
|---|---|---|---|
| Benign | Cyst & Adenoma | 70 | 113 |
| | Dermoid Cyst | 40 | |
| | Solid Tumor | 3 | |
| Borderline | | 9 | |
| Malignant | | 36 | |
| Total | | 158 | |

December 1979, 149 patients were admitted to the Departme-nt of Gynecology at Okayama University Hospital. After USG on them, laparotomies were performed and histopatholo-gical diagnoses were confirmed.

We examined unilateral ovarian tumor in 140 cases and bilateral ovarian tumors in 9 cases, totaling 158 tumors. Table 1 shows the number of tumor at each histological group of 158 tumors for which histological diagnosis was performed. Those cases with ovarian tumor were divided into 3 groups, namely benign, borderline and malignant groups(Table 1).

The echo patterns obtained from ovarian tumors were analyzed in the sixteen items having 2 to 4 categories respectively(Table 2).

The incidence in each category were assessed by each group with benign, borderline and malignant tumors accord-ing to the histological diagnosis(Table 2). The results obtained were statistically analyzed by the use of Fisher's exact or chi-squere test to find which item was more effective for discrimination among three groups. Signifi-cant bias in distribution was found in following items: 1) size of mass (the longest diameter), 5) smoothness of bou-ndary echo of mass, 7) thickness of capsel echo on cystic part, 9) presence of septum echo interior cystic part, 12) presence of solid part and its size compared with whole mass size, 13) shape of solid part and 16) presence of as-cites. In summary, both borderline and malignant groups had tumors with more than 15 cm in diameter, irregular boundary, cystic part with thick or ununiformly thick cap-sel and septum, irregular shaped solid part and ascites.

QUANTIFICATION ANALYSIS AND WEIGHTED SCOREING SYSTEM

Based on the above analysis those seven items, which were deemed important, were arrenged into six new items (Table 3) and their categories were given tentative

Table 2. The items and their categories of echo pattern

| Item | Category |
|---|---|
| 1) Size of mass (the longest diameter) | a) Shorter than 5 cm<br>b) 5 to 10 cm<br>c) 10 to 15 cm<br>d) Longer than 15 cm |
| 2) Uni- or bilateral | a) Unilateral<br>b) Bilateral |
| 3) Distinguishability from uterus | a) Separate from uterus<br>b) Border on uterus<br>c) Undistinguishable |
| 4) Continuity of mass wall (boundary) | a) Continuous<br>b) Uncontinuous |
| 5) Irregularity of mass wall (boundary) | a) Smooth mass wall<br>b) Irregular mass wall |
| 6) Cystic part in the mass | a) Present<br>b) Lack |
| 7) Thickness of cystic wall | a) Thin<br>b) Thick<br>c) Unequal |
| 8) Protrusion of cystic wall into the inside | a) Present<br>b) Lack |
| 9) Septum in the cystic part | a) Present<br>b) Lack |
| 10) Thickness of septum in the cystic part | a) Thin<br>b) Thick<br>c) Unequal |
| 11) Inner echo amplitude of cystic part | a) Echo free<br>b) Low amplitude |
| 12) Solid part and its size compared with the whole mass | a) Lack<br>b) Present but smaller than 1/3 of whole mass<br>c) Present and 1/3—2/3<br>d) Present and larger than 2/3 |
| 13) Shape of solid part | a) Smooth shape<br>b) Irregular shape |
| 14) Homogeneity of solid part | a) Homogenous<br>b) Heterogenous |
| 15) Echo amplitude of solid part | a) High amplitude<br>b) Middle amplitude |
| 16) Ascites | a) Present<br>b) Lack |

and number of tumors at each category

| Histological Group | | | | |
|---|---|---|---|---|
| Benign | Borderline | Malignant | Total | |
| 18 | 0 | 0 | 18 | * |
| 49 | 0 | 14 | 63 | |
| 28 | 3 | 12 | 43 | |
| 18 | 6 | 10 | 34 | |
| 103 | 9 | 28 | 130 | |
| 5 | 0 | 4 | 9 | |
| 41 | 6 | 11 | 58 | |
| 66 | 1 | 20 | 87 | |
| 4 | 1 | 2 | 7 | |
| 96 | 6 | 27 | 129 | |
| 17 | 3 | 9 | 29 | |
| 42 | 6 | 31 | 79 | * |
| 71 | 3 | 5 | 79 | |
| 107 | 9 | 35 | 151 | |
| 6 | 0 | 1 | 7 | |
| 61 | 2 | 14 | 77 | * |
| 10 | 0 | 5 | 14 | |
| 34 | 6 | 15 | 55 | |
| 20 | 4 | 7 | 31 | |
| 85 | 4 | 27 | 116 | |
| 25 | 6 | 17 | 48 | * |
| 80 | 2 | 17 | 99 | |
| 9 | 0 | 4 | 13 | |
| 5 | 1 | 5 | 11 | |
| 11 | 5 | 8 | 24 | |
| 90 | 6 | 29 | 125 | |
| 17 | 3 | 6 | 26 | |
| 49 | 0 | 0 | 49 | * |
| 26 | 5 | 14 | 45 | |
| 23 | 3 | 12 | 38 | |
| 15 | 1 | 10 | 26 | |
| 29 | 1 | 4 | 34 | * |
| 35 | 8 | 32 | 75 | |
| 25 | 1 | 9 | 35 | |
| 39 | 8 | 27 | 74 | |
| 24 | 3 | 8 | 35 | |
| 40 | 6 | 28 | 74 | |
| 0 | 2 | 4 | 6 | * |
| 108 | 7 | 28 | 143 | |

non-weighted scores(Table 4). To determine the relation between two groups with external standard, by the separated quantity, the Quantification Analysis No. 2 developed by Hayashi as a statistical procedure, is presently available. Based on the benign, borderline and malignant groups as external standard, the quantification analysis was conducted using the tentative scores given as the separated quantity. And normalized scores, that are weighted scores, were given to each category of the item(Table 5).
Statistically it was found that the smaller of the

Table 3 Summerizing method of valuable items for analysing by Quantification No. 2

| Statistically valuable items by chi-square test | Selected items used for analysis by Quantification No.2 |
|---|---|
| 1) Size of mass | 1) Size of mass |
| 5) Irregularity of mass wall | 2) Irregularity of mass wall |
| 6) Mass with cystic part | |
| 7) Thickness of cystic wall | 3) Cystic part and the thickness of its wall |
| 9) Septum in cystic part | 4) Septum in cystic part |
| 12) Solid part and its size | |
| 13) Shape of solid part | 5) Solid part and its shape |
| 16) Ascites | 6) Ascites |

Table 4 Non-weighted scores of 6 items

| Longest Diameter | — 5 cm | 4 | Cystic Part (−) | | 4 |
| | 5—10 cm | 3 | (+) & Septum (−) | | 3 |
| | 10—15 cm | 2 | | Thin | 2 |
| | 15— cm | 1 | | Thick or Unequal | 1 |
| Boundary | Smooth | 2 | Solid Part (−) | | 3 |
| | Rough | 1 | (+) & Shape | Regular | 2 |
| | | | | Irregular | 1 |
| Cystic Part (−) | | 4 | | | |
| (+) & Wall | Thin | 3 | Ascites | (−) | 2 |
| | Thick | 2 | | (+) | 1 |
| | Unequal | 1 | | | |

185

Table 5 Normalized score, its range and partial correlation coefficient of 6 items analysing by Quantification No. 2

| Item & Category | Normalized Score | Range | Partial Correlation Coefficient |
|---|---|---|---|
| Longest Diameter    — 5cm<br>5—10cm<br>10—15cm<br>15— cm | 20.85<br>5.77<br>- 6.07<br>-13.07 | 33.92 | 0.325 |
| Boundary   Smooth<br>Rough | 4.79<br>- 6.02 | 10.81 | 0.161 |
| Cystic Part   (-)<br>(+) Wall   Thin<br>Thick<br>Unequal | 20.27<br>3.98<br>4.78<br>- 5.70 | 25.97 | 0.161 |
| Cystic Part   (-)<br>(+) Septum   (-)<br>Thin<br>Thick or<br>Unequal | -11.70<br>3.98<br>5.61<br>- 9.29 | 17.31 | 0.184 |
| Solid Part   (-)<br>(+) Shape Regular<br>Irregular | 20.78<br>13.07<br>-19.61 | 40.39 | 0.494 |
| Ascites   (-)<br>(+) | 2.41<br>-51.96 | 54.37 | 0.325 |

normalized scores were suggesting the higher possibility with which the tumor was in malignant or borderline group. The category indicating the highest possibility of tumor in borderline or malignant group included ascites(+), followed by the solid part with irregular forms and more than 15 cm in length. The category an intensive possibility of tumor in benign group was found to have less than 5 cm in length and solid part(-) or cystic part(-).

In each item the range of normalized scores as well as partial correlation coefficient were dirived(Table 6). It was indicated that the larger these figures were the more important for discriminating two groups, and the presence of irregular shaped solid part and ascites were very significant.

The sum of the normalized scores of each item is called as a total normalized score. The distribution of the total normalized score in the three groups, which were histologically classified, is shown in Figure 1.

Figure 1 Graph for discrimination between benign group and borderline and malignant groups

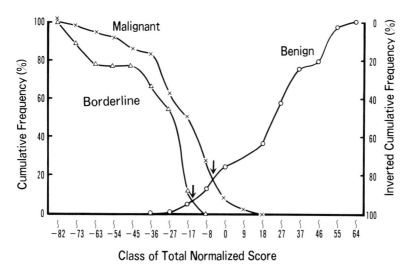

Table 6 Classification of zone by normalized score and its distribution

| Zone | Class of Normalized Score | Histological Group | | |
| --- | --- | --- | --- | --- |
| | | Malignant | Borderline | Benign |
| Malignant | — -17 | 50.0% | 88.9% | 5.3% |
| Doubtful | -16 — 9 | 47.2% | 11.1% | 23.9% |
| Benign | 10 — | 2.8% | 0.0% | 70.8% |

The smaller of total normalized score indicates that the tumor is in borderline or malignant group. Based on the distribution of total normalized scores at each group, the total normalized scores were divided into three zones. Table 6 shows the class of total normalized scores in each zone and incidence (frequency) in each group as well.

PROSPECTIVE USE OF WEIGHTED SCORING SYSTEM

Among the patients on whom USG was performed during the period of January 1980 to October 1981, we observed ovarian tumor in 56 cases which histological diagnosis was confirmed. The relationship in 56 cases between the histological group and the zones classified by echo pattern weighted scoring system is shown in Table 7. In the his-

187

Table 7 Result of prospective study

| Zone | Histological Group | | | Total |
| --- | --- | --- | --- | --- |
| | Malignant | Borderline | Benign | |
| Malignant | 8(88.9%) | 0 | 8(17.0%) | 16(28.6%) |
| Doubtful | 1(11.1%) | 0 | 9(19.1%) | 10(17.9%) |
| Benign | 0 | 0 | 30(63.8%) | 30(53.6%) |
| Total | 9 | 0 | 47 | 56 |

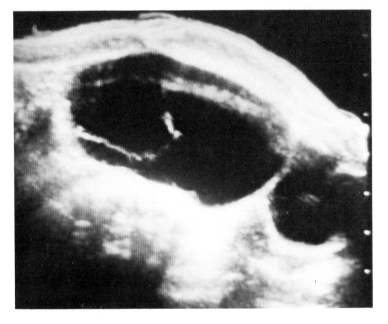

Figure 2 Median longitudinal section of mucinous cystadenoma and data printed out

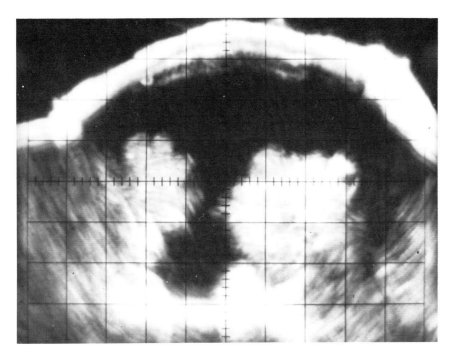

```
#ｸﾀﾞﾉﾀﾞ  ﾋﾞｮﾛ 56ｻｲ  ｶﾞｲﾗｲNo 6379  ｴﾝｲﾝNo  63  USG-No 1068
ﾘｮｳｿｸﾃｲ---ﾋﾀﾞﾘ
Size of Mass  8.0 x  6.0 x  6.5 Cm  Volume  312 Cmﾘｯﾎﾟｳ
Uterush  ﾊﾟﾄﾚﾃｲﾙ
ﾍｷ ﾉ ﾚﾝｿﾞｸｾｲ(+)
ﾍｷ ﾌﾃｲ
Cystic Part(-)
Solid Part(+)  2/3ﾖﾘﾖﾘｼﾞｮｳ
                ﾀｲﾅｲ ﾌﾃｲ
                #ﾋﾞﾙ
                high amplitude
Ascites(+)
Total Score(Root 1)=-63.2 Probability of BENIGN=  0% -MALIGNANT ZONE-
Total Score(Root 2)=001.6 Probability of MALIG.= 84% BORDERLINE=16%
ﾘｮｳｿｸﾃｲ---ﾐｷﾞ
Size of Mass  6.0 x  6.0 x  6.0 Cm  Volume  216 Cmﾘｯﾎﾟｳ
Uterush  ﾊﾟﾄﾚﾃｲﾙ
ﾍｷ ﾉ ﾚﾝｿﾞｸｾｲ(+)
ﾍｷ ﾌﾃｲ
Cystic Part(-)
Solid Part(+)  2/3ﾖﾘﾖﾘｼﾞｮｳ
                ﾀｲﾅｲ ﾌﾃｲ
                #ﾋﾞﾙ
                high amplitude
Ascites(+)
Total Score(Root 1)=-63.2 Probability of BENIGN=  0% -MALIGNANT ZONE-
Total Score(Root 2)=001.6 Probability of MALIG.= 84% BORDERLINE=16%
```

Figure 3 Transverse section of bilateral cystadenocarcinoma and data printed out

tologically malignant group, 88.9% came under the malignant zone and the rest 11.1% was classified as doubtful zone.
There was no falsely benign case.

In the cases with benign tumor, those in malignant or
doubtful zone accounted for 36.1% which showed a higher
percentage than 25% obtained in the retrospective study.

This showed the available limit of the present procedure.

We have used USG for body imaging in our department as the first choice. In such case indicating doubtful or malignant zone, X-ray computed tomography(CT) as well radioisotope scintigraphy with Ga-67 were performed. Though the findings by the combination use of those, the cases with 100% malignant and 97% benign tumor undertook operations, all of them being diagnosed correctly before operation(6). From the result, it is probable that an infectious ovarian tumor may erroneously be diagnosed as a malignant ovarian tumor.

The ultrasound examination room of our department is equiped with microcomputer. The findings of USG are immediately printed out as shown in Figure 2-3. The programs including patient's name, year, outpatients, inpatients and ultrasound numbers, and 16 ultrasound findings with questions and answers, are stored on a minifloppy disk. Immediately after these questions, these answers together with total (normalized) score, probability of benign tumor and zone are printed out. While it was not stated in this report, the computer program also involves Root 2 procedure for discrimination of malignant group from borderline group, and the results are printed out simultaneously.

In the weighted scoring system, it is necessary to read the findings from all the categories. It is considered therefore that diagnosis of ovarian tumor may be possible in a fair and accurate manner at any organization equipped with ultrasound to be handled by less skilled staffs or many other persons.

REFERENCES

1. Takeuchi, H., Kawamata, C., Sugie, T., Kobayashi, T. (1977): In: Excerpta Medica International Congress Series No. 436 Recent Advances in Ultrasound Diagnosis, P. 113. Editor: A. Kurjak, Omsterdam-Oxford.
2. Saiki, M., Takayanagi, M., Matsushita, M., Sogawa, T., Yoshida, A., Kono, M., Shimada, H.(1980): JSUM Proceedings, 34, 333.
3. Kurimura, Y., Koh, D., Hashizume, T., Yamaoka, T., Hamaoka, H., Hanioka, Y., Hisamatsu, K., Fujiwara, A. (1980): JSUM Proceedings, 37, 115.
4. Sekiba, K., Fukumoto, S., Akamatsu, N., Hirai, T., Lin, T.T., Niwa, K., Tsubota, N.(1981): JSUM Proceedings, 38, 495.
5. Sekiba, K., Fukumoto, S., Fujita, T., Akamatsu, N.: In: Excerpta Medica International Congress Series, in press.
6. Akamatsu, N., Fukumoto, S. Fujita, T., Hirai, T., Nishi, M., Niwa, K., Sekiba, K.(1981): Acta Obstet. Gynecol. Jap., 33, 2338(Abst.).

# CHORIOCARCINOMA: POSSIBLE PREVENTION BY EARLY ULTRASOUND DIAGNOSIS OF BLIGHTED OVA

A. Kurjak, P. Jouppila, F. Rusinović and V. D'Addario

*Ultrasonic Centers, Zagreb, Oulu and Bari*

One of the greatest mysteries of placentate reproduction is the mechanism whereby the trophoblastic inversion of the maternal host is halted. On the occasions when this fails the consequences may be hydatidiform mole or chorionic carcinoma.

Hydatidiform mole occurs with a frequency of the order of 1:2,000 or 3,000 pregnancies in Europe and 1:200 or 300 in Asia. Choriocarcinoma follows a mole in from 2 to 17% of cases and is the principal mortality risk.

Until recently it was contended that chorionic carcinoma was a uniformly fatal condition and that, if a patient said to have the condition survived, the diagnosis was in error (1).

The advent of chemotherapeutic agents active against trophoblast,and in particular the folic-acid antagonist Methotrexate, has revolutionised the situation. Despite this achievement, however, there are still many problems in this area.

## GENESIS OF HYDATIDIFORM MOLE

Much has been written and said about the pathology and classification of trophoblastic neoplasia, all to very little purpose.

MARCHAND suggested in 1895 that 50% of chorionic carcinomas were preceeded by hydatidiform mole, 25% by normal pregnancy and the remaining 25% by abortion or ectopic pregnancy (2).

In their remarkable paper published in 1940 HERTIG and EDMONDS considered that the lesion is due to retention of a blighted ovum, with cessation of the villous stromal circulation and continued secretory activity of the trophoblast, nourished by the maternal blood; this results in varying degrees of hydrops and trophoblastic proliferation (3).

On the other hand PARK and his team regarded it as a primary trophoblastic abnormality (4).

Hydropic change has long been recognised as a common finding in abortuses, but it was HERTIG and EDMONDS (1940) who carried out the first formal study into the nature of the change. They examined products of conception in 1027

191

cases, together with 74 hydatidiform moles. There was a
high incidence of "blighted ova" in products of spontaneous abortion; hydropic change was present in 67% of those
abortions with 'pathological' ova and in only 12% of those
with 'non-pathological' ova (3).

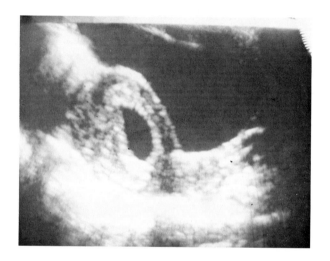

Fig. 1A.   Case 1.   9 weeks gestation.   Empty sac.

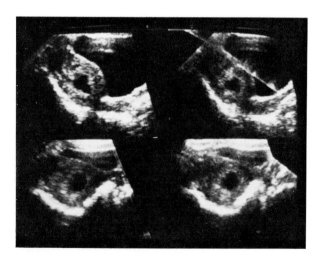

Fig. 1B.   One week later size of gestational sac decreased.

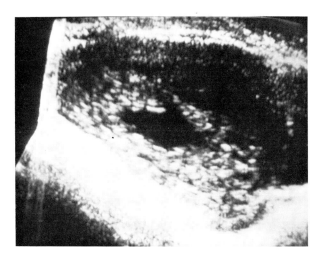

Fig. 1C. 13 weeks gestation. Longitudinal scan; enlarged uterus filled with vesicular tissue and poorly formed gestational sac.

In their view the sequence of events in the genesis of a hydatidiform mole commences at about five weeks' menstrual age, when the fetal circulation is normally established. The death or blighting of the embryo results in failure of establishment of the fetal villous blood vessels, and in the presence of actively secreting trophoblast, fluid accumulates within the villous stroma, since there is no mechanism for its removal. It is suggested that the trophoblastic hyperplasia is due to stretching by the swollen villi. The authors regard the classical hydatidiform mole as one end of a continuous spectrum of hydatidiform degeneration, the other end of which is characterised by the spontaneous abortion with only occasional hydropic villi. In support of this concept they reported that pathological ova were aborted at an average menstrual age of 10 weeks, non-pathological ova at 15.5 weeks, transitional moles at 16.5 weeks, and classical hydatidiform moles at 17.5 weeks.

Since these pioneer papers there has been little progress to further explain the nature of trophoblastic disease. Recently an excellent paper was published by HANDO and his team. Their careful study consisted of 391 early spontaneous abortions and of 230 cases of hydatidiform mole (5). Like HERTIG and EDMONDS their work showed that blighted ova accompanied the initial or early stages of hydatidiform mole in more than two-thirds of the cases, but most of them were expelled from the uterus by 10 or 11 weeks of gestation, before they had sufficient time to develop into macroscopic hydatidiform moles. When for unknown reasons expulsion of the conceptus is delayed, the so-called molar changes develop. They concluded that hydatidiform mole is a special type of missed abortion, the final stages in the natural history of a retained and growing blighted ovum.

From all of these quoted papers it seems that hydatidiform mole is a special type of delayed expulsion of the blighted ovum, and not a tumour in itself. The logical conclusion therefore would be that by early diagnosis of blighted ovum and consequent interruption of pregnancy one could prevent the development of hydatidiform mole and perhaps of choriocarcinoma.

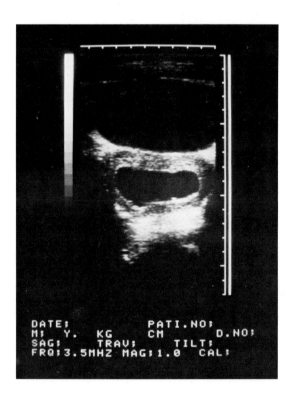

Fig. 2A. Case 2. Empty gestational sac at 8 weeks amenorrhea.

194

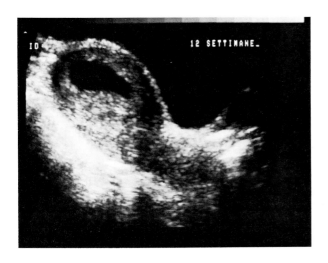

Fig. 2B.The same case at 12 weeks.

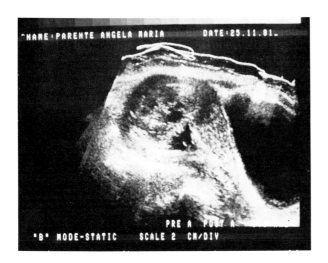

Fig. 2C. Typical molar appearance

DIAGNOSIS OF BLIGHTED OVA

Blighted ova constitute about one half of spontaneous abortions and ultrasound is the method of choice in the diagnosis and assessment of this form of early pregnancy failure (6). The information obtained by the biochemical and histopathological evaluations can help in better understanding of functional and structural capacities of blighted ova but are of no practical value in early and reliable diagnosis if ultrasound can be used (7).

Observations concerning the commonness of chromosomal anomalies in abortive tissues have elucidated this problem in quite a new and reasonable way. LAURITSEN found 60% of chromosomal anomalies in the tissues of spontaneous abortions. Most of these were autosomal translocations (8). According to POLAND and MILLER, frequency of chromosomal anomalies in blighted ova was 50% (9). Diagnosis has now been greatly enhanced by the introduction of the real-time ultrasonic machine.

Our own results have shown that with real-time ultrasonography the diagnosis of blighted ova was possible in 100% of the cases studied after two examinations, one week apart (10). The distinction between normal pregnancy and a blighted ovum is simple enough and these vital results are available for use immediately.

On the other hand, the value of the biochemical determination of different trophoblastic markers seems to be relatively limited in the diagnosis of blighted ova.

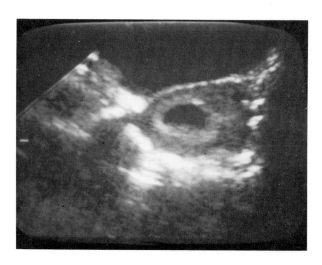

Fig. 3A. Case 3. Gestational sac at 8 weeks.

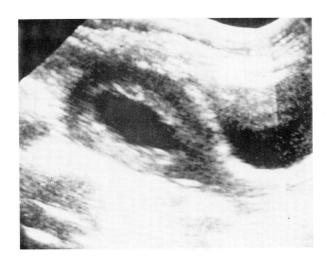

Fig. 3B. 10 weeks; size of gestational sac increased; no fetus.

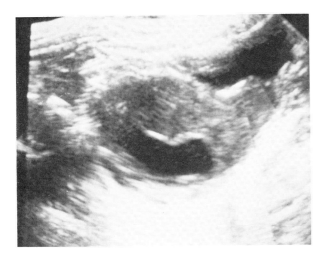

Fig. 3C. 12 weeks - enlarged uterus containing poorly formed gestational sac.

In a collaborative study performed at the universities of Zagreb and Oulu, ultrasonic, biochemical and histopathological investigations of the blighted ovum have been carried out. The first group consisted of 300 blighted ova detected by ultrasound only. The final diagnosis was made after the first examination in 70% of the cases, after 2 examinations in 28% of cases and after 3 examinations in 2% of the cases. Group II consisted of 65 blighted ova in which the serum level of progesterone, estradiol and human chorionic gonadotropin were measured. Using serum HCG, prognostic prediction could be made correctly in only 71% of all the cases in the group. Group III consisted of 72 patients in which histopathological examination of the uterine contents was performed. In 17% of the cases, evaluation of the primary pathological features was uncertain and they were scored as likely pathological ova (7).

The very high incidence of molar pregnancy in primary blighted ova which were retained in utero for several weeks demonstrates the importance of early and reliable diagnosis of the blighted ovum. Even HERTIG noticed that when a blighted ovum fails to abort and is retained and survives, it eventually becomes a true hydatidiform mole.

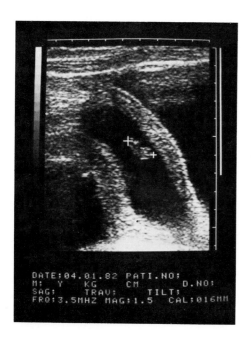

Fig. 4A. Case 4. Large gestational sac at 11 weeks with rudiment marked by crosses.

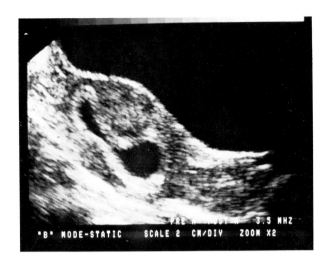

Fig. 4B.  The same case one week later.

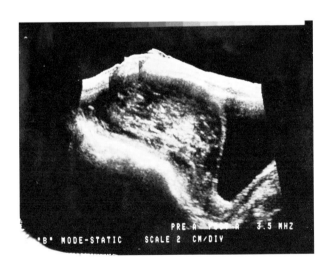

Fig. 4C.  Obvious molar appearance at 14 weeks.

According to HORMANN and LEMTIS such a blighted ovum is usually aborted between the 11th and 13th week; a hydatidiform mole is usually expelled after the 16th week (11). Our results correspond very well with these early findings. Indeed, both authors observed an obvious decrease of molar pregnancy after successful early detection of blighted ova.

Finally, couples with blighted ova are high risk patients in subsequent pregnancies because of a very high incidence of genetic disease. Therefore, such patients should receive genetic counselling and adequate control in further pregnancies.

OUR RECENT STUDIES

Having noticed in a previous study that 7 out of 13 cases originally diagnosed as blighted ova later developed into hydatidiform moles after 17 weeks, we carried out a systematic study of this problem in Zagreb. One member of our team (F.R.) examined over a two-year period 404 pregnant women with bleeding in the first 14 weeks of pregnancy. In 300 (74%) of investigated patients fetal life was confirmed and 90% of patients had successful pregnancy outcomes. Among the remaining 104 patients (26%) without any signs of fetal life, the most common form of early pregnancy failure was blighted ovum. There were 53 blighted ova or 51% of all the early pregnancy failures. The incidence of blighted ovum in patients with bleeding in early pregnancy (404) was 13%. Here it should be stressed that this is the incidence in patients who bled in the first trimester but not in the general obstetric population. In the latter group the incidence will be higher because a significant proportion of blighted ova come to ultrasonography without signs of bleeding.

In this group we had 8 cases of hydatidiform mole originally discovered as blighted ova but interrupted before 14 weeks. There was only one case of late hydatidiform mole, and this woman came for the first ultrasound examination at 13 weeks amenorrhea where typical molar changes were found. In the last four years there have been no cases of choriocarcinoma among the over 17,000 women examined by ultrasound. Some illustrative cases are shown in Figures 1-6.

CONCLUSION

Controversy still surrounds the pathogenesis of hydatidiform mole. The most fundamental problem was and still is the discovery of the ultimate cause of abnormal trophoblastic growths. It is to be hoped that the geographic, demographic, biochemical and immunological studies currently being undertaken will elucidate the etiological mechanism and that it will prove to be one against which practical remedial action can be taken. In the meantime, the risk will be minimised by measures to achieve early diagnosis. Until recently diagnostic ultrasound was used for the detection of this disease in the first and second trimester. However, in 1977 we noticed and illustrated the possibility that hydatidiform mole may arise from a blighted ovum.(12-14). This was reconfirmed by our subsequent collaborative study (7). Present studies also support our previous observations as 8 moles have been detected during the first trimester.

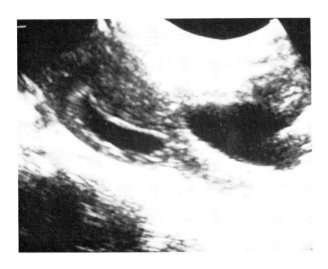

Fig. 5A. Case 5. Gestational sac at 9 weeks; no fetus.

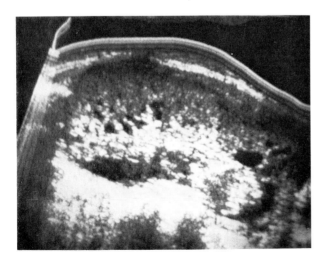

Fig. 5B. Typical hydatidiform mole with multiple cystic structures.

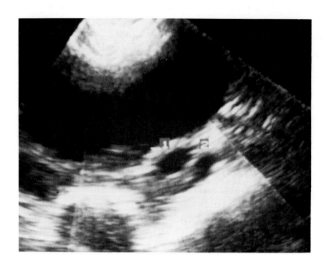

Fig. 6A.  Case 6.  Two empty gestational sacs at 6 weeks
gestation.

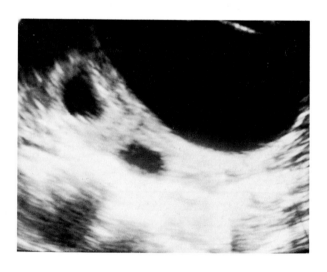

Fig. 6B.  The same empty sac at 9 weeks.

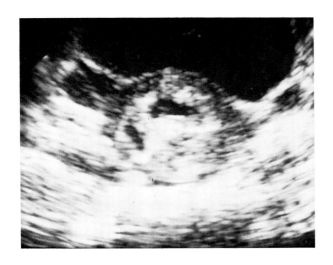

Fig. 6C. The size of both sacs decreased. Obvious trophoblastic reaction. Hydatidiform mole was confirmed microscopically.


    The risks of hydatidiform mole fall into three cate-
gories: (a) immediate from haemorrhage, sepsis or prae-
clampsia, (b) from the occurrence of molar metastasis,
and (c) from subsequent development of chorionic carcinoma.
    In a recent report by WITTMANN et al (15) four such
cases have been described. Ultrasonic findings in cases
of first trimester molar pregnancies have also been evaluated (16). In three cases the intrauterine picture was similar to the typical findings in missed abortion or incomplete abortion. According to the figures in the latter paper it is possible that the authors were demonstrating the
intermediate stage between blighted ovum and final hydatidiform degeneration. If the hypothesis proposed from these
cases can be confirmed in wider studies, it is possible that
by early ultrasonic detection of blighted ova and by active
management (evacuation) of these doomed pregnancies, the
number of cases of gestational trophoblastic disease can
be diminished (17,18).

REFERENCES

1. Edmonds, H.W. (1953): Ann. N.Y.Acad.Sci. 80,196.
2. Marchard, F. (1895): MSCHR. Geburtsch.Gynäk. 1,413,513.
3. Hertig, A.T., Edmonds, H.W. (1940): Arch.Pathol.20,260.
4. Park, W.W. (1959): Ann.N.Y.Acad.Sci. 80,99.
5. Hando, T., Hirogami, T. et al. (1980): In: Gynecology and Obstetrics, Tokyo, October 25-31,1979, pp.548-554. Editors: Shoichi Sakamoto, Shimpei Tojo, Tetsuja Nakayama.
6. Hertig, A.T., Sheldon, W.H. (1943): Ann.Surg. 117,596.
7. Kurjak, A., Jouppila, P. (1981): J. Foetal Med. 1,54.
8. Lauritsen, J.G. (1976): Acta Obst.Gyn.Scand.Suppl.52,18.
9. Poland, P.J., Miller,J. R. (1973): In: Proceedings of the Symposium on Les Accidents Chromosomiques de la Reproduction, Paris, September 1973, pp.111-118.
10. Kurjak, A., Kirkinen, P. Banović, I., Rukavina, B. (1980): In: Recent Advances in Ultrasound Diagnosis, pp.139-143, Editor: A. Kurjak, Excerpta Medica, Amsterdam.
11. Hormann, G., Lemtis H. (1965): Die Menschliche Placenta, Urban und Schwarzenberg, Munchen-Berlin.
12. Kurjak,A. (1977): In: Recent Advances in Ultrasound Diagnosis, pp. 209-223, Editor: A. Kurjak, Excerpta Medica, Amsterdam.
13. Kurjak, A., Latin, V. (1979): Acta Obstet.Gynecol.Scand. 58,153.
14. Kurjak,A. (1980): In: Progress in Medical Ultrasound, p.125, Editor: A. Kurjak, Excerpta Medica, Amsterdam.
15. Wittman, B.K., Fulton, L., Cooperberg, P.L., Lyons, E.A., Miller, C., Shaw, D. (1981): J.Clin.Ultrasound 9,153.
16. Woodward, R.M., Filly, R.A., Callen, P.W. (1980): Obstet. Gynecol. 55,31.
17. Jouppila, P. (1982): In: Progress in Medical Ultrasound 3, Editor: A. Kurjak, Excerpta Medica, Amsterdam.
18. Jouppila, P., Huhtaniemi, I., Tapanainen, J. (1981): Obstet.Gynecol. 55,42.

# ULTRASOUND FOR THE DIAGNOSIS OF RETROPERITONEAL CANCER

Barry B. Goldberg

*Division of Ultrasound and Radiologic Imaging, Department of Radiology, Thomas Jefferson University Hospital, Philadelphia, PA, U.S.A.*

When reviewing the importance of ultrasound in the diagnosis of various abnormalities, its multiple uses in the retroperitoneum become readily apparent (1,2). The retroperitoneum, extending from the diaphragm down into the pelvis, contains many structures. It contains such organs as the kidneys and adrenals, as well as lymph nodes, nerves, muscles, blood vessels, and fat. The pancreas and portions of the bowel, although also retroperitoneal, will not be discussed in this chapter. Ultrasound evaluation of the urinary bladder and prostate, however, will be reviewed. In the limited amount of space available, it would be impossible to cover, in depth, all possible retroperitoneal cancers. Emphasis will be placed in several major areas such as the kidneys, adrenals, and urinary bladder. To give the readers some concept of how frequently ultrasound is used in the retroperitoneum, a review of the world literature for only the past two years has found over 300 articles written relating to this area. The anatomy of the retroperitoneum is well established (3). An understanding of the various compartments has been provided by the use of computerized tomography, and has allowed the ultrasonographer to further understand the best approaches for obtaining the maximum information in these areas. While ultrasound in the retroperitoneum can be used to diagnose many non-cancerous abnormalities, this chapter will deal specifically with its usefulness in tumor diagnoses and differentiation.

IMAGING TECHNIQUES

Ultrasonic evaluation of the retroperitoneum, no matter what structure, has become surprisingly routine, at least for the initial surveying of the areas of interest. As a result, rather than discussing techniques individually under each area, i.e. renal, adrenal, etc., this portion of the chapter will serve to provide basic technique information.

For examination of the right retroperitoneum, that is, right kidney and adrenal, the patient is first positioned supine. Longitudinal scans are then obtained, using the liver through which to transmit the sound beam.

A simple linear and then sector scans under the rib cage will usually result in an excellent image, particularly if the patient has suspended respiration and an appropriately focused transducer has been utilized. Longitudinal scanning of the right kidney is best obtained starting medially so that the vena cava is initially visualized. This is the best approach for evaluation of masses posterior to the vena cava, which includes the medial extension of the right adrenal gland. Succeeding slices, usually at 1 cm. intervals, should extend to the lateral edge of the abdomen until the kidney has been completely imaged. Transverse scans of the right retroperitoneum are then obtained by relying on the longitudinal information to designate the appropriate levels. Scanning usually starts from the level of the xyphoid at 1 cm. intervals to at least the level of the iliac crest. If there is concern about abnormalities in the lower abdomen and pelvis, the transverse scans can be extended downward over the iliac crest into the pelvis. While, on occasion, the left retroperitoneum can be seen from a supine approach, this is rare due to the interposition of bowel gas from the stomach, small bowel, and colon. Thus, for examination of the left retroperitoneum, the best images are usually obtained with the patient in a decubitus position. This approach can also be used on the right to provide additional information not available with the supine approach. The patient is positioned left side up, and a transducer moved in a longitudinal direction, incrementing from posterior to anterior. Of course, in this relatively small space between the costal margin and iliac crest, sector scanning often produces the best images. With this approach, not only the kidney but also the spleen and adrenal gland can be seen. The degree of angulation, from posterior to anterior or anterior to posterior, will vary depending on the variations in position of the kidney. The more posterior skin approach with anterior angling of the transducer appears to be the best for visualization of the adrenal (4). A similar approach can be utilized for the right side. When the coronal longitudinal scanning is complete, then a series of transverse images can be obtained, using the information provided by the initial longitudinal images to determine the levels at which to start and end the scanning.

Finally, if insufficient information is obtained from either the right supine or either right or left decubitus views, a prone approach can be utilized. With the patient prone, scans both longitudinal and transverse can be obtained of the renal area. This approach, although initially the most common approach for ultrasound visualization of the retroperitoneum, has decreased in importance due to the realization that the often dense back muscle and nearby bone, as well as aerated lung and iliac crest, often prevents adequate visualization. However, it should be realized that if a comparison between

kidneys is desired on the same image, only the prone
transverse approach can provide that information.  This
can be helpful when there is a problem in terms of sound
transmission through a mass in order to compare one side
to the other.

The lower abdomen and pelvis are best scanned when
the patient is supine.  The decubitus and prone views are
not effective due to the iliac wings preventing penetration of the ultrasonic beam.  The initial longitudinal
imaging should be midline in order to be sure that the
urinary bladder is adequately filled.  Scanning is then
continued laterally to the right and left, usually at
1 cm. intervals.  After completion of this initial sequence, transverse images are obtained, starting at the
pubic bone and moving in a cephalad direction.  By angling
the transducer caudad, imaging of the deep pelvis is often
improved for such structures as the prostate and seminal
vesicles.  For evaluation of the distal ureters, oblique
longitudinal scanning angling toward the bladder trigon
is the best approach.

It should be pointed out that various types of both
static and real-time equipment can be effectively used in
the evaluation of most of the retroperitoneum.  The only
limitations are the lateral decubitus views where equipment capable of sector scanning has an advantage.  For
the lower abdomen, however, sector, linear, and static
B-scan equipment can all be effectively utilized.

RENAL

The usefulness of ultrasound in the evaluation of
renal masses, both in adults and children, has been well
established (5) (Fig. 1A&B).  In adults a mass is usually
found on routine intravenous urography.  The next step is
an ultrasound examination using the techniques described
previously in this chapter.  Not only is ultrasound able
to anatomically image the area in question, but it is also
able to determine its size and internal structure.  In
those cases where a mass is palpated, usually in children,
ultrasound has also assumed its role as a primary evaluator, being used in some cases even before intravenous
urography.  With increasing utilization of ultrasound for
many areas within the abdomen and pelvis, it is not unusual to detect renal or other retroperitoneal masses while,
for instance, an examination of the liver is being performed.  With increased use of real-time equipment, the
relative speed with which the abdomen can be surveyed has
lead to an increased pickup of incidental retroperitoneal
masses.

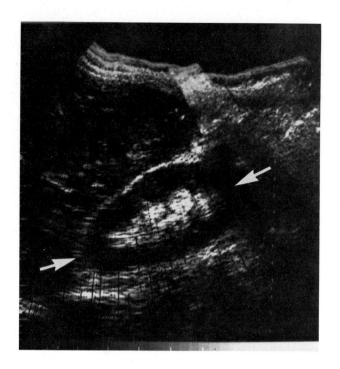

Figure 1A. Longitudinal supine ultrasonogram demonstrates
a normal right kidney (arrows). Note normal contour as
well as normal central hilar echogenicity and well-defined
capsule.


    The ability of ultrasound to detect and differentiate
masses has been established with an overall accuracy of at
least 95% (6). This ability is one that allows the differentiation of a mass into its fluid or solid components.
Of course, a mass that is echo-free and has good through
sound transmission is characteristic of a cyst, while one
that has multiple internal echoes with attenuation of the
sound, resulting in weak distal wall echoes, is typical
of a solid mass. This statement, however, is a simplistic
one since there are a number of possible combinations of
these two, resulting in complex (mixed) type masses.

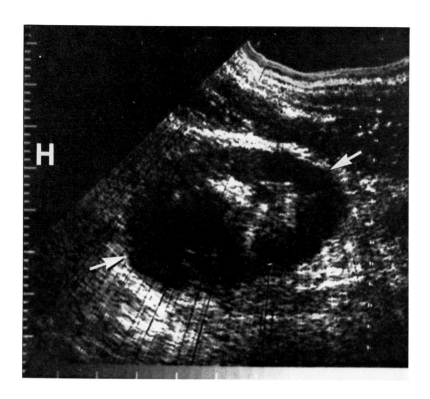

Figure 1B. LOngitudinal decubitus ultrasonogram of the left kidney (arrows) demonstrates enlargement of the upper pole with distortion of the echogenic central hilar region due to a renal cell carcinoma of the upper pole. (H - direction of head)

While a small percentage of renal tumors are benign in nature, it must be assumed that whenever a solid ultrasound pattern is obtained that the renal mass is malignant. The most common renal tumor, of course, is renal cell carcinoma (hypernephroma). Attempts have been made to try to use ultrasound to differentiate the type of renal tumor by its ultrasound characteristics (7). The differing ultrasonic patterns of solid masses are related to a number of factors. The variation in echogenicity, with some tumors tending to be of relatively low internal echogenicity and others high, is related to the number of internal interfaces and the acoustic differences between tissues making up the mass. Thus, the factors that tend to produce increased echogenicity include hypervascularity, diffuse fibrous or fatty tissue, non-uniformity of tissue, as well as areas of hemorrhage and necrosis (Fig. 2). All of these factors will tend to produce in-

terfaces and therefore an increase in the overall echogenicity. Other factors, such as the presence of calcification, can also cause increased echogenicity (Fig. 3).
Thus, tumors that have small areas of punctate calcification or hemorrhage, fatty-fibrous tissues (as is typical
of angiomyolipomas), and/or hypervascularity often have
an overall increased echogenicity. While attempts have
been made to correlate the degree of echogenicity with
one particular factor, such as hypervascularity, this has
not been proven to be specific (8). In most cases, a
number of factors must be present for the degree of echogenicity to be significantly greater than average.

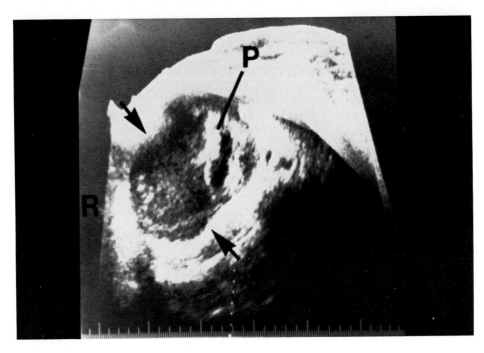

Figure 2. Transverse supine ultrasonogram of the right
kidney shows a mass (arrows) with moderate internal echogenicity extending laterally from the right kidney.
There is associated dilatation of the renal pelvis (P).
(R - right)

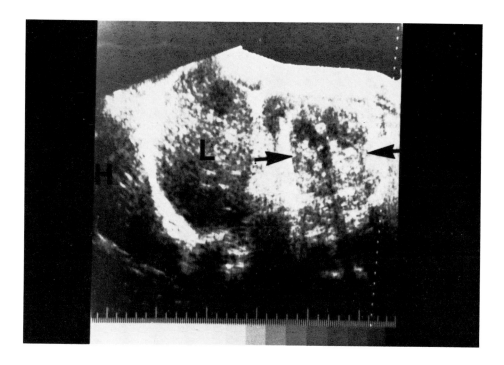

Figure 3. Supine longitudinal ultrasonogram delineates a large echogenic mass (arrows) with focal bright echoes and distal acoustic shadowing in some areas due to scattered calcification. Biopsy under ultrasonic guidance was positive for renal cell carcinoma. (L - liver)


The reverse can be said for tumors that are hypoechogenic. They generally have weak back walls due to attenuation but yet have relatively few internal echoes. These types of tumors tend to be of uniform cell type, sparse vascularity, and have no significant areas of hemorrhage or necrosis. Like the echogenic type tumors, multiple factors are usually involved. The most common types of tumors are lymphomas and other infiltrative processes, as well as metastatic tumors. While one can use these characteristics to suggest the possibility of one or another type of tumor, such as angiomyolipoma with highly echogenic tumors or lymphoma with weakly echogenic tumors, it has been shown that hypernephromas may have any of these characteristics and, therefore, must always be included in the differential diagnosis (Fig. 4).

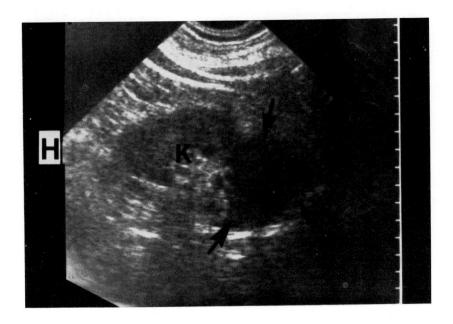

Figure 4. Longitudinal decubitus ultrasonogram of the left kidney shows an irregular weakly echogenic mass (arrows) arising from the lower pole, which proved to be a renal cell carcinoma. (K - kidney)

Finally, tumors may be mixed or complex in nature. Generally, these masses have fairly good through transmission with varying internal echogenicity (Fig. 5). This type of pattern can be produced by any tumor which undergoes necrosis or hemorrhage as well as by abscesses and hematomas. The clinical history is usually sufficient to aid in making a specific diagnosis possible, i.e. necrotic tumor, abscess, or hematoma.

Tumors may occur not only within the parenchyma but also within the central renal hilar region. These types of tumors tend to be transitional cell carcinomas. They may have various ultrasonic patterns. There may be difficulty on routine intravenous urography to differentiate this from a central cyst or non-opaque calculi. Ultrasound is helpful in making the appropriate differential diagnosis.

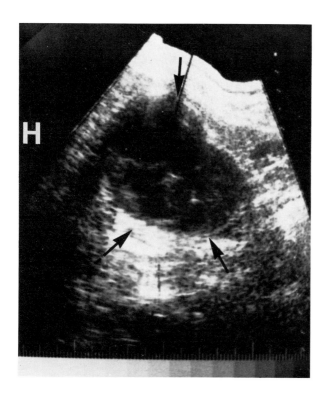

Figure 5. Decubitus longitudinal ultrasound of the left kidney shows a large mass (arrows) distorting the entire kidney. The tumor can be seen to be complex in nature with irregular internal echoes and distal acoustic enhancement, indicating its higher than average fluid content. At surgery, this was proven to be a necrotic renal cell carcinoma.

Infiltrative tumors, such as leukemia, may present as bilateral large kidneys with the parenchyma having an overall decreased echogenicity (9). Lymphoma may also present as an infiltrative process or as separate tumor masses. In the pediatric age group leukemic infiltrate is not uncommon, but the most common renal mass, particularly in early childhood, is Wilms' tumor. This usually presents as an echogenic mass with relatively good through sound transmission, particularly in the larger tumors, due to areas of hemorrhage and/or necrosis (10).

Besides the identification and differentiation of renal tumors, ultrasound has been used effectively to evaluate for tumor spread, both locally and at a distance. Thus, whenever a renal tumor is detected ultrasonically, the renal vein and inferior vena cava should be examined. In some cases tumor thrombus may be seen extending through the renal vein into the vena cava (11). The entire course of the vena cava should be examined since the tumor thrombus can even extend up into the right atrium. The typical pattern is that of an area of increased echogenicity within the vein (Fig. 6). The adjacent retroperitoneum should be carefully examined to evaluate for local extension as well as spread to regional lymph nodes. It should be pointed out, however, that for regional extension and disruption of tissue planes, computerized x-ray tomography often provides the most information (12).

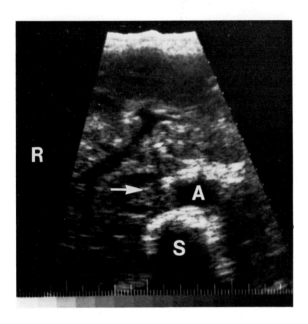

Figure 6. Transverse supine ultrasonogram of the mid-abdomen shows the vena cava to contain internal echoes (arrow), consistent with the diagnosis of a tumor thrombus from a previously demonstrated right renal tumor. Note relatively echo-free aorta (A). (S - spine)

Finally, ultrasound has been used for serial evaluation in those cases where a renal tumor is being treated nonsurgically. Changes in size as well as internal texture can be observed ultrasonically during or after treatment due to necrosis and/or hemorrhage. Dramatic changes in size have been reported in cases of lymphoma and leukemia. Serial evaluation has also been used effectively in children to visualize the remaining kidney in cases of Wilms' tumors since bilaterality is not infrequent. Some

214

syndromes that have increased incidents of renal tumors also lend themselves to serial ultrasound evaluation, reducing the need for repetitive intravenous urography.

ADRENAL

While computerized x-ray tomography has established itself, in most instances, as the primary modality in the evaluation of adrenal abnormalities, when a suprarenal mass is detected on routine intravenous urography, ultrasound can be used effectively to confirm and differentiate the mass (13). Thus, using the previously described techniques for adrenal imaging, ultrasound can determine the size and position of suprarenal masses as well as their internal characteristics. When no mass can be detected ultrasonically, this certainly does not exclude its presence. The ability of ultrasound to visualize the normal adrenal gland is limited and thus minimal tumors can be easily missed. Longitudinal imaging is usually the best approach to separate the adrenal mass from the kidney (Fig. 7A&B). However, if a separation is not seen between the mass and kidney, one may well have to rely on arteriography to establish the origin of such a tumor (Fig. 8).

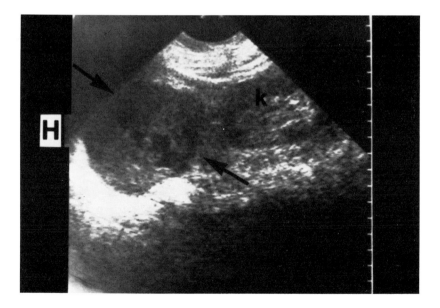

Figure 7A. Decubitus longitudinal ultrasonogram demonstrates a large suprarenal mass (arrows) having multiple internal echoes and distal enhancement indicating it to be complex in nature. Note that it is separate from the kidney (K).

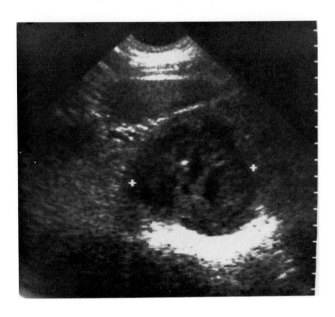

Figure 7B. Transverse ultrasonogram of the same mass confirms its complex nature (+'s used to determine size). This proved to be a pheochromocytoma.


Ultrasound has very low pathologic specificity; while it can identify the presence of a mass and its internal characteristics, these alone are not enought to allow for tumor identification. Many different types of tumors can occur in this region, including adenomas, carcinomas, pheochromocytomas, neuromas, as well as tumors of metastatic origin. Non-organ related tumors such as those arising from the muscles, fibrous tissue, fat, or blood vessels, usually sarcomatous in nature, can also present in the suprarenal region. All these masses are either solid or complex in nature, depending on the presence of hemorrhage and/or necrosis. The reasons for the differences in internal echogenicity are the same as described earlier in the renal section of this chapter. Adrenal tumors may be bilateral and, in fact, the most common are metastatic in origin. Many different primary tumors can metastasize to the adrenals. These can become quite large since they may be relatively asymptomatic and in this region are difficult to palpate. Only indirect evidence by displacement of the kidneys may lead to even the suggestion that the adrenals may be involved with tumor. Some tumors, such as pheochromocytomas, of course, may present with a specific clinical history, such as label hypertension, to draw attention to this area. While many similar tumors may occur in the pediatric age group, one of the most common is neuroblastoma, which may have scattered calcifications and therefore have areas of increased echogenicity. As in the adult, ultrasound can be used effectively to evaluate for spread, both contiguous and distant. For instance, in neuroblastomas, the liver should be carefully examined ultrasonically since metastasis to this organ from this tumor is not infrequent.

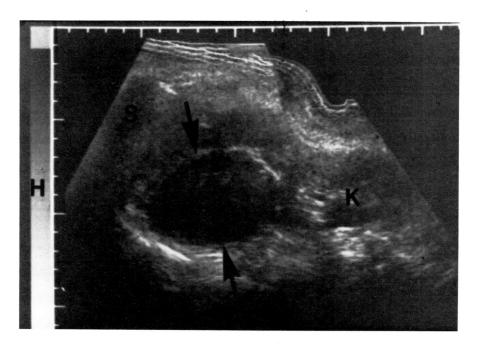

Figure 8. Longitudinal decubitus view demonstrates a weakly echogenic suprarenal mass (arrows) located between the spleen (S) and kidney (K). The origin of the mass was confirmed by arteriography. This proved to be an adrenal metastasis. The opposite adrenal was also involved.


NONSPECIFIC RETROPERITONEAL TUMORS

As stated previously, retroperitoneal tumors may arise from any of the tissues, i.e. fat, fibrous, muscle, and vessel. Thus, sarcomatous tumors from various structures can be detected ultrasonically. The site of origin of the masses, of course, cannot usually be delineated. The most common nonspecific retroperitoneal tumor is a liposarcoma. This can present as a highly echogenic tumor due to the multiple interfaces arising from the mix-

217

ture of fat, fibrous tissue and blood vessels usually present. However, when such tumors undergo necrosis or hemorrhage, they present with a complex pattern (14).

The relationship of the tumors to adjacent structures can often be delineated. This is particularly true for the kidney where its displacement by a retroperitoneal mass can often be detected (Fig. 9A&B). It should be pointed out that retroperitoneal tumors can extend into the anterior abdomen and, if invasive in nature, may encase the adjacent blood vessels.

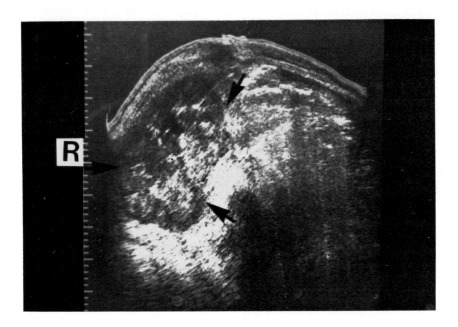

Figure 9A. Supine transverse ultrasonogram shows evidence of large irregular echogenic mass (arrows) that appears to be arising from the retroperitoneum and extending anteriorly. The site of origin of this tumor could not be completely identified from this image.

Among the most common retroperitoneal tumors are those arising in lymph nodes (Fig. 10). These can be either metastatic or primary, most commonly lymphoma, lymphosarcoma, or Hodgkin's disease. Differentiation between the types of lymphomas cannot be made ultrasonically. The nodes may be visualized individually or may become confluent and present as a large mass. These masses may be purely retroperitoneal in nature and displace the vena cava and aorta anteriorly. These types of tumors may sometimes be difficult to separate from adrenal or other types of retroperitoneal masses. However, classical extension of nodes in the para-aortic region resulting in a draping weakly echogenic mass anterior to the aorta and vena cava will usually suggest the appropriate differential diagnosis. The response to treatment can easily be followed ultrasonically. While negative ultrasound findings will not exclude the presence of involved lymph nodes, once enlarged nodes have been identified, ultrasound can be used to serially follow the response to treatment, whether it be chemotherapy or radiation. The identification of nodes within the pelvis is not as readily made ultrasonically as those that are para-aortic or retro-caval. Pelvic lymph node involvement is best demonstrated by tomography. The determining factors are often the size of the patient, with obese patients being more easily evaluated with computerized tomography and thin and pediatric patients with ultrasound.

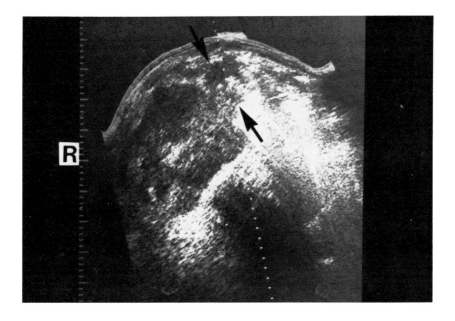

Figure 9B. At another level, the tumor can again be seen on the right but, in addition, the right kidney has been identified (arrows) being displaced anteriorly and medially. This helped to confirm that the mass was a retroperitoneal tumor, which proved to be a liposarcoma.


Ultrasound has been used effectively as a guide to the biopsy of tumors (15). This has been particularly true in the kidney and to a lesser extent with other retroperitoneal masses. Once a mass has been determined to be solid ultrasonically, a specially modified static or real-time transducer can be utilized to guide a needle into place for a successful biopsy. Ultrasound is not only able to determine the exact pathway, away from vital structures, but also the exact depth for placement of the needle. With this ultrasonic technique, the pathway of the needle can be easily determined and an echo from the region of the tip of the needle usually recorded, allowing for a more accurate guidance than with other non-ultrasonic techniques. Thus, as a result, ultrasonic biopsy techniques have become a routine procedure in the staging of many retroperitoneal tumors.

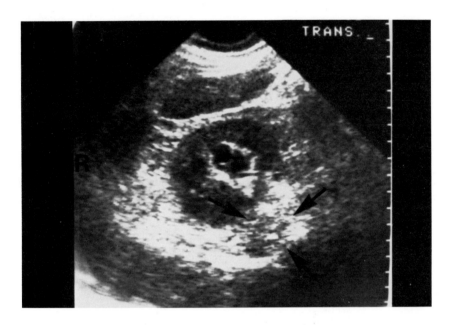

Figure 10. Transverse supine ultrasonogram at the level of the right kidney shows mild hydronephrosis. Just posteriorly there is seen to be an irregular mass (arrows) which proved to be an enlarged lymph node. Other lymph nodes were also identified in the para-aortic region in this patient who was known to have lymphoma.


PELVIS

Retroperitoneal tumors can arise within the pelvis, such as neurogenic tumors, as well as those arising from any of the tissues (i.e. muscle, nerve, fat, etc.). Teratomatous masses, for instance, arising from the region of the sacrum projecting into the pelvis, have also been delineated ultrasonically. In the female patient, differentiation of ovarian tumors from retroperitoneal masses may sometimes be difficult. In fact, unless the ovaries can be identified separately, one often has to assume that tumors are ovarian in origin. If the mass displaces the rectosigmoid anteriorly, then a diagnosis of a retro-peritoneal tumor rather than ovarian can be made. Using ultrasound water enema techniques or x-ray barium enema such differentiation may be made (12).

URINARY BLADDER

The urinary bladder, when distended with urine, acts as a good window through which to transmit the ultrasonic beam and to visualize structures deep within the pelvis. However, this same distended bladder can itself be evaluated ultrasonically to determine the presence of tumor (16). Bladder tumors will usually present as filling defects within the normally echo-free fluid. They may be polypoid or sessile in nature. Those that protrude into the bladder from the wall are easy to define. Those that tend to spread along the surface may be a little more difficult to delineate but, usually with adequate distention, the tumor mass can be imaged (Fig. 11). Evaluation of spread into the muscle and beyond is more difficult ultrasonically. Sometimes the muscle wall of the bladder can be identified as a thin hypoechogenic region just beneath the more echogenic mucosa. When this is not present, the possibility of invasion must be considered (17). As far as evaluating extension beyond the bladder wall, computerized x-ray tomography is more advantageous and usually can demonstrate invasion of the adjacent tissue planes.

PROSTATE

The prostate has been successfully evaluated ultra-sonically by a variety of approaches (18). The standard abdominal approach is similar to that described for evaluation of the urinary bladder. However, endoscopic and perineal approaches have been used. To obtain an image of the prostate perineally, the transducer is moved between the scrotum and anus with the sound beam directed in a cephalad direction. For an endoscopic image, a special probe containing a transducer must be placed within the rectum. Both static and real-time endoscopic approaches have been used to obtain images (Fig. 12). An endoscopic probe has also been developed that can be placed within the bladder via the urethra (19). With this approach, both bladder and prostatic tumors can be evaluated. These endoscopic approaches show promise in being able to identify smaller tumors than with the routine external approaches. Work is in progress attempting to differentiate benign prostatic disease from malignant. With these endoscanning approaches it is possible to record the prostatic capsule to determine if it is intact. Of course, if there is a break in the capsule, this is a much more serious problem (20). As with bladder tumors, extensive spread is best evaluated with computerized x-ray tomography.

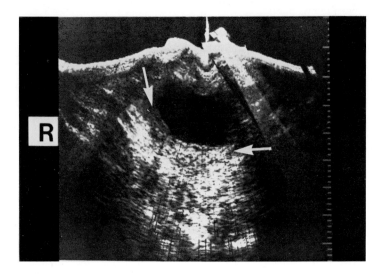

Figure 11. Supine transverse ultrasonogram of the urinary bladder demonstrates a posterior wall sessile tumor (arrows), which proved to be an extensive infiltrating transitional cell carcinoma.

In conclusion, ultrasound has established itself as a primary evaluator for many tumors of the retroperitoneum. It is used routinely whenever a mass is palpated or found on routine urography. While it has not yet been proven useful for specific tumor identification, it can determine the size and location of many retroperitoneal masses as well as delineate their internal structure, i.e. fluid versus solid content. Beyond that, ultrasound has also been used successfully to evaluate response of these tumors to treatment. The advantages as well as limitations of ultrasound in the evaluation of retroperitoneal tumors have been reviewed. In the future, special techniques including endoscanning may well lead to the ability to identify specific tumors.

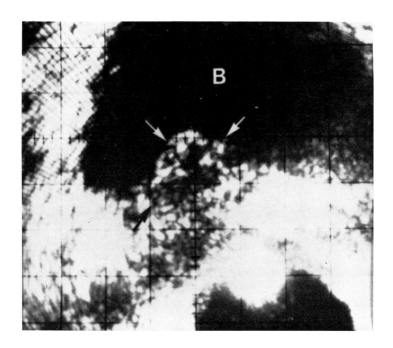

Figure 12. Transverse ultrasonogram obtained using an
endoscopic rectal approach shows the urine-filled bladder
(B), within which can be seen protruding from the posterior wall an irregular echogenic mass (arrows), which at
surgery proved to be an invasive prostatic carcinoma.
(Courtesy of Bruno Squassabia, Verona, Italy)

REFERENCES

1.  (1977). Abdominal Gray Scale Ultrasonography.
    Editor: B.B. Goldberg. John Wiley & Sons, Inc.,
    New York.
2.  (1981). Ultrasound in Cancer. Editor: B.B. Goldberg.
    Churchill Livingstone, Inc., New York.
3.  Meyers, M.A. (1976): Dynamic Radiology of the
    Abdomen. Springer-Verlag, New York.
4.  Sample, W.F. (1977): Radiology 124:463-469.
5.  Watanabe, H., Holmes, J.H., Holm, H.H. and Goldberg,
    B.B. (1981): Diagnostic Ultrasound in Urology &
    Nephrology. Igaku-Shoin, Tokyo, Japan.
6.  Lingard, D.A. and Lawson, T.L. (Dec. 1979): The
    Journal of Urology, 122:724-727.
7.  Ladwig, S.H., Jackson, D., Older, R.A. and Morgan, C.L.
    (Feb. 1981): Urology, (17)2:204-209.
8.  Coleman, B.G., Arger, P.H., Mulhern, C.B., et. al.
    (1980): Radiology, 137:757-765.

9.  Kaude, J.V. and Lacy G.D.  (1978):  J. Clin. Ultra-
    sound, 6:295-382.
10. Gates, G.F., Miller, J.H. and Stanley, P.  (June
    1980):  The Journal of Urology, Vol. 123:916-920.
11. Pussell, S.J. and Cosgrove, D.O.  (1981):  British
    Journal of Radiology, 54:866-869.
12. Levine, E., Lee, K.R. and Weigel, J.  (Aug. 1979):
    Radiology, 132:395-398.
13. Sample, W.F. and Sarti D.A.  (1978):  Radiology,
    128:377-383.
14. Chung, W.M., Ting, Y.M. and Gagliardi, R.A.  (1978):
    J. Clin. Urol., 6:266-267.
15. Goldberg, B.B., Pollack, H.M. and Kellerman, E.
    (April 1975):  Radiology, 115:167-170.
16. McLaughlin, O.S., Morley, P., Deane, R.F., et. al.
    (Feb. 1975):  Brit. J. Urol., 47:51.
17. Itzchak, Y., Singer, D. and Fischelovitch, Y.
    (July 1981):  Journal of Urology, Vol. 126,
    pp. 31-36.
18. Resnick, M.I.  (1980):  Semin. Ultrasound, 1:69-79.
19. Nakamura, S. and Nijima, T.  (1980):  J. Urology,
    124:341-344.
20. Watanabe, H., Igari, D., Tanahashi, Y., et. al.
    (Nov. 1975):  J. Urol., 114:734.

# ULTRASOUND OF RETROPERITONEUM PRIMITIVE TUMORS

N. Frédéric, M. D'Hondt, H. Claes, F. Van Droogenbroeck and R. Potvliege

*Department of Radiology, University Hospital Brugmann, Brussels, Belgium*

An analysis of 25 cases of primary retroperitoneal tumors is presented. Among these very rare tumors, sarcoma is the most common histopathologic type.

Their characteristics are that they attain large size before clinical manifestations, displacing adjacent organs and causing pressure phenomena.

Differential diagnosis are discussed.

Echographic patterns are related to the macroscopic features of the different tumors and a "most probable diagnosis" can be proposed.

## MATERIAL AND METHODS

These three last years (September 78 - February 82) 7.200 echografies of the upper abdomen were performed.

Most of them were performed with a compound digital scanner (Picker 80 L), 20 % with a real time imager (A.T.L. - A.D.R. - TOSHIBA).

2.25 MHz and 3.5 MHz transducers were used unless limited by patient size.

## RESULTS

37 retroperitoneal tumors were found : 10 metastatic carcinomas, 2 metastatic carcinomas of unknown origin invading spine and retroperitoneal space, 25 primary retroperitoneal tumors.

The histopathologic repartition of those primary tumors is : 8 of lymphatic origin, 9 embryonal tumors, 8 "primary" retroperitoneal tumors.

More details are shown on table 1.

TABLE 1. Repartition of 25 primary retroperitoneal tumors :

| | | |
|---|---|---|
| 8 lymphatic | : | 1 Hodgkin |
| | | 2 Lymphosarcomas |
| | | 4 lymphomas |
| 9 embryonal | : | 1 seminoma |
| | | 5 ovarian adenomas |
| | | 3 ovarian carcinomas |

8 "primary" retroperitoneal :

> 3 Leiomyosarcomas
> 2 Liposarcomas
> 1 Rhabdomyosarcoma
> 1 Teratoma

All cases were proved by surgery, biopsy or autopsy.

DISCUSSION

The retroperitoneum extends from the twelfth rib and vertebra, to the base of the sacrum and the iliac crest (17) (15). The space contains loose areolar tissue through which pass the I.V.C., aorta, ureters, renal vessels, gonadal vessels and numerous lymphnodes (17). This potentially large space allows primary and metastatic tumors to grow silently before clinical signs and symptoms appear (17).

There are often general symptoms or disturbances due to compressions : thromboses, paresthesias, hydronephroses, edema, ascitis (19).

The use of ultrasound, following a clinical examination and simple plain film, is essential to determine size, extension and contents of a mass and from what organ the mass arises (16).

In the upper abdomen, Whalen describes two different situations :

1. The mass is high situated and displaces the spleen posteriorly, the kidney inferiorly.

2. The tumor arises from the lower part of the upper abdomen and displaces pancreas and stomach anteriorly, duodenum inferiorly, kidney posteriorly and laterally (19).

The following classification (TABLE 2) excludes lesions of the kidney, ureter, adrenal gland, liver, pancreas, duodenum, spleen or metastatic tumor secondary to neoplasm arising elsewhere.

TABLE 2.  Classification of Retroperitoneal Neoplasms :

I. Tumors of mesodermal origin :

> A. Highly differentiated
> 1. Liposarcoma
> 2. (Lipoma)
> 3. Leiomyosarcoma
> 4. (Leiomyoma)
> 5. Rhabdomyosarcoma
> 6. Fibrosarcoma
> 7. (Hemangioma)
> 8. Hemangiopericytoma

B. Poorly differentiated
   1. Mixed tissue tumor-mesenchymoma
   2. Spindle-cell sarcoma-undifferentiated sarcoma
   3. Myxoma

II. Tumors of neural origin :

   A. Sympathetic nervous system
      1. Neuroblastoma
      2. (Ganglioneuroma)
      3. (Paraganglioma, inactive)
      4. Paraganglioma, active-extra-adrenal pheochromocytoma

   B. Neural sheath
      1. (Neurofibroma)
      2. (Neurilemoma)
      3. Schwannoma

III. Tumors of lymphatic origin

   A. Lymph nodes
      1. Hodgkin's disease
      2. Reticulum cell sarcoma
      3. Lymphosarcoma
      4. Giant follicle lymphoma

   B. Lymph vessels
      1. (Lymphangioma)

IV. Tumors of embryonic rest tissue

      1. (Teratoma)
      2. Testicular and ovarian tumors
      3. Chordoma
      4. (Wolffian cyst)

---

Primary tumors of the retroperitoneum are very rare, exception made of neoplasms arising in the kidney, adrenal gland and lymph nodes.
However, the designation of "retroperitoneal tumors" usually qualify tumors arising outside these structures (17).
If we except tumors arising from the lymph nodes, the most frequent are the liposarcoma, the leiomyosarcoma and the embryonal carcinoma (fibrosarcoma and rhabdomyosarcoma being exceptional) (17) (TABLE 3).

TABLE 3. Relative frequencies of malignant R.P. tumors:
(17)

| | |
|---|---|
| - Lymphosarcoma | 19 % |
| - Liposarcoma | 13 % |
| - Leiomyosarcoma | 11 % |
| - Hodgkin | 10 % |

| - <u>Embryonal carcinoma</u> | 9 % |
| - Hemangiopericytoma Sympathicoblastoma | 7 % |
| - Metastatic carcinoma of unknown origin | 5 % |
| - Teratoma | 2.3 % |
| - Rhabdomyosarcoma | 2 % |
| - Fibrosarcoma | 1.5 % |

(A.P. Stout-serie of 265 tumors)

Herein, we attempt to correlate previously descri-bed aspects of primary retroperitoneal tumors with the sonographic patterns.

1. LIPOSARCOMA : has lobulated fatty masses and a "brain-tissue" - like aspect. It is often multiloculo-ted and has a predilection for the perirenal area (17). In our cases, the fatty zones are very echogenic (1) and polilobulated. There was compression of the adjacent kidney (Fig. 1) (12).

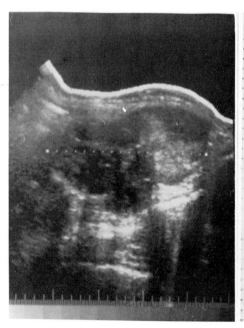 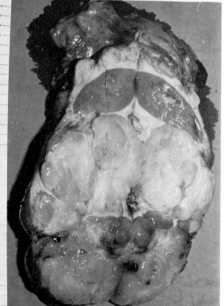

Figure 1.a : Ultrasound of a pararenal liposarcoma

1.b : Surgical specimen

Bilobulated fatty masses, compressing and displacing the kidney superiorly (very echogenic on U.S.)

2. LEIOMYOSARCOMA : is the second most frequent sarcoma in this area (8). It is often encapsulated and has a particular tendency to undergo massive cystic degeneration when occuring in this region (13).
Ultrasound will easily show encapsulated and heterogenous mass containing transonic liquid zones (Fig. 2).

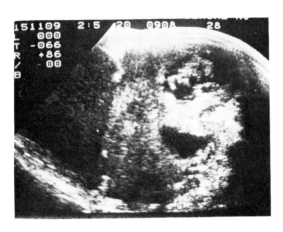

Figure 2 : Ultrasound of a leiomyosarcoma of the left hypochondrium : see numerous liquid zones of cystic necrosis, in an otherwhile heterogenous mass (longitudinal scan).

3. RHABDOMYOSARCOMA : arises from the muscle, contains hemorrhagic zones, which are transonic on ultrasound (17).

4. FIBROSARCOMA : is one of the rarest tumors and has some common features with the leiomyosarcoma encapsulated with central necrosis (10).

5. NEUROGENIC TUMORS : are not nearly so common as in the mediastinum (17). Pheochromocytoma is a soft cellular, often hemorrhagic mass, sharply defined by a thin capsule.
SCHWANNOMA is a large homogenous, nodular and well encapsulated mass (it is less often cystic or necrotic) (Fig. 3).

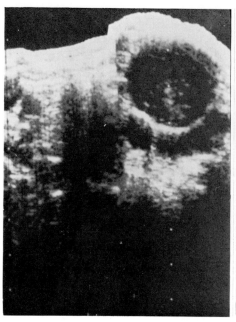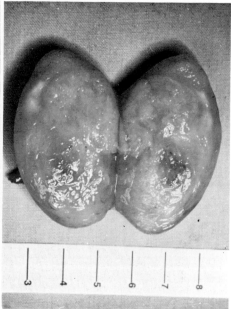

Fig. 3.a : U.S. of a cervical schwannoma shown for
its particular homogenous consistency
(transverse scan).

3.b : Surgical removed specimen.

6. GERMINAL CELL TUMORS : are mainly represented by
the benign teratoma (5). It is often large and cystic.
Ovarian and testicular tumors can also occur in this
location and have the same aspect (18).

We have an example of seminoma (arising from cystic
degeneration of a cryptorchidian testicle) which has
exactly the same aspect as an ovarian carcinoma.
(Aberrant germinal tissue frequently is found in the
retroperitoneum and may undergo malignant change in this
location) (4) (Fig. 4).

Melicow reported the ratio of malignant to benign
retroperitoneal tumors to be 4 to 1, based on his study
of 162 cases (14), so that we have to be very carefull
in the diagnosis of benign lesion even if it looks
purely cystic and well encapsulated.

Bree correlated histologic type of 28 mesenchymal
sarcomas with their sonographic pattern, and found four
different ultrasonic patterns : hyperechoic masses with
anechoic zones, hyperechoic masses with central fluid-
filled zones, homogenous hyperechoic masses, homogenous
hypoechoic masses. He concluded that the presence of a
large mass with necrosis should strongly suggest the
possibility of sarcoma (2) (11).

230

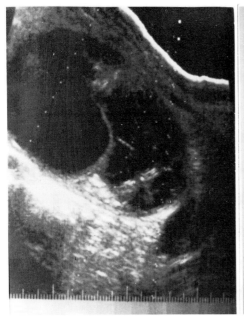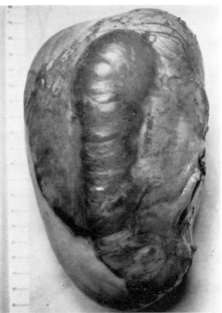

Fig. 4.a : U.S. of a seminoma (from a cryptorchidian
testicle) : a well encapsulated cystic
lesion (long scan).

4.b : Surgical removed specimen.

The differential diagnosis are : any cystic of
mixed lesion of the retroperitoneum (pancreas, kidney,
omentum, spleen ...) (9).

- Tumors of the gastro-intestinal tract, which have
a kidney like appearance.

- Fluid collections (abscesses, hematomas, aneurysm)
which are particular transonic and have a lentiform
shape (20).

- Retroperitoneal fibrosis which can be characterized by a solid homogenous transonic mass compressing
the great vessels (6).

- Tumors arising from spine and bony pelvis, which
are seen on the plain film (3).

CONCLUSION :

Ultrasound can often reveal the size, shape, anatomical relations of retroperitoneal masses, assessing
the extent of disease and, sometimes, it can give an
indication of consistency (cystic, solid, fatty, necrotic, calcified) (11) and a more precise etiology, or a
"most probable" diagnosis between liposarcoma, leiomyosarcoma and germinal tumors, which are the most frequent
(7).

231

REFERENCES

1. BEHAN M. : The echographic characteristics of fatty tissues and tumors. Radiology, 129 : 143-151,1978

2. BREE R. : The grey scale sonographic appearance of intraabdominal mesenchymal sarcomas. Radiology, 128 : 193-197, 1978

3. DE SANTOS L.A. : Ultrasonography in tumors arising from the spinde and bony pelvis. Amer. J. Roentgenol., 129 : 1061-1064, 1977

4. DUNCAN R.E. : Diagnosis of primary retroperitoneal tumors. J. Urol., 117 : 19-23, 1977

5. ENGEL, R.M., ELKINS, R.C. and FLETCHER, B.D. : Retroperitoneal teratoma ; review of the literature and presentation of an unusual case. Cancer 2:1068-1973, 1968.

6. FAGAN Ch.J. : Retroperitoneal fibrosis : ultrasound and C.T. features. Amer. J. Roentgenol., 133 : 239-243, 1979.

7. FREDERIC N. : Ultrasound of the retroperitoneal space - J. Belge Radiol., 64 : 63-73, 1981.

8. GOLDEN T. and STOUT, A.P. : Smooth muscle tumors of the gastrointestinal tract and retroperitoneal tissues, Surg. Gynecol. Obstet. 73 : 784-810, 1941.

9. Hsu-Chong Ych. Ultrasonography and Computed Tomography in the diagnosis of Homogenous Masses. Radiology 123 : 425-428, 1977.

10. KAHN, L.B. : Retroperitoneal xanthogranuloma and xanthosarcoma (malignant fibrous xanthoma) Cancer 31 : 411-422, 1973.

11. KARP W. : Retroperitoneal Sarcoma : U.S. and Angiographic evaluation. Brit. J. Radiol. 53 : 525-531, 1980.

12. KIM G. : Contralateral displacement of abdominal viscera by a retroperitoneal liposarcoma : ultrasonic demonstration. J. Clin. Ultrasound, 5 : 117-120, 1977.

13. LUMB, G. : Smooth-muscle tumors of the gastrointestinal tract and retroperitoneal tissues presenting as large cystic masses. J. Pathol. Bacteriol 63:139-147, 1951

14. MELICOW, M.M. : Primary tumors of the retroperito-
    neum : a clinicopathologic analysis of 162 cases ;
    review of the literature and tables of classifica-
    tion.  J. Int. Coll. Surg.  19: 401, 1953.

15. MEYERS A. MORTON : Dynamic R-diology of the abdomen.
    Normal and pathologic anatomy. Springer-Verlag,1976.

16. SENECAIL B. : Apport de l'échographie dans l'explo-
    ration des masses géantes de l'abdomen chez l'adulte.
    Ann. Radiol., 23 : 41-44, 1980.

17. SOUT A.P. : Tumors of the retroperitoneum, mesentery
    and peritoneum.  Atlas of tumor pathology.
    Armed Forces Institute of Pathology, Washington,1954.

18. WALSH J.W. : Prospective comparison of U.S. and
    C.T. in the evaluation of gynecologic pelvic masses.
    Am. J. Roentgenol. 131 : 955-960, 1978.

19. WHALEN J.P. : Vector principle with differential
    diagnosis of abdominal masses : the left upper qua-
    drant.
    Amer. J. Roentgenol., 113 : 104-118, 1971.

20. WICKS, J.D. : Ultrasonic characterization and diffe-
    rential diagnosis of abdominal fluid collections.
    Contemporary Diag. Rad. Vol. 4, n° 4, 1981.

# DIAGNOSTIC IMPACT OF ULTRASONOGRAPHY IN THE EVALUATION OF RETROPERITONEAL TUMORS PRESENTING AS PALPABLE MASSES

Giorgio Rizzatto, Massimo Bazzocchi, Mario Maffessanti, Franca Brizzi, Claudio Ricci and Ludovico DallaPalma

*Institute of Radiology, University of Trieste, Trieste, Italy*

Retroperitoneum may be involved by a varied group of tumours.These are often large enough to be detected on physical examination (6).This finding may urge the physician to resort imaging methods that would confirm the clinical finding and provide additional information on the site of origin,the actual extent and the nature of the mass.
We report our experience in the ultrasonographic evaluation of 43 retroperitoneal tumours collected from a retrospective review of proven cases of abdominal lesions presenting as palpable masses.

MATERIALS AND METHODS

During a five-year period (March 1977 – January 1982) we have studied 133 patients affected by 136 proven retroperitoneal lesions presenting as palpable masses.At surgery or autopsy 43 of these masses turned out to be of tumoural nature;their distribution is summarized in table 1:

TABLE 1.Distribution of 43 retroperitoneal palpable tumours

| | | | |
|---|---|---|---|
| Renal................13 | | | |
| Suprarenal.......... 9 | primary tumours | 8/9 | |
| | secondary tumours | 1/9 | |
| Pancreatic.......... 4 | | | |
| Retroperitoneal.....17 | primary tumours | 12/17 | |
| | secondary tumours | 5/17 | |

All the patients were studied using dynamic scanners with both linear and mechanical sector transducers;digital grey-scale contact B-scanners were also used whenever possible.Dynamic scanning may be used alone in pediatric studies or whenever the poor condition of the patient makes access difficult for the static scanner.In all the other cases it provides additional information on organs movement and preliminarily suggests the best scanning

planes.On the other hand static scanning may allow some
better informations on both the internal structure and
the topographic location of these masses.

RESULTS

Renal tumours
     All the 13 renal tumours presenting as palpable mas-
ses were correctly identified also with regards to their
organ of origin.Neoplasms more frequently involved the
right kidney (10/13);in 5 cases the tumour affected all
the kidney.
In 6 out of 9 cases renal vein and/or IVC thrombosis were
defined;this task was possible only for tumours originating from the right kidney.Secondary liver deposits could
also be demonstrated;on the other hand fascial infiltration could only be suspected and ultrasonography also
failed to assess suprarenals or limphnodes involvement in
every case subsequent CT examinations or surgery gave positive results.
All the tumours showed irregular margins and a solid echo
pattern;echogenicity was always higher than normal parenchyma,often inhomogeneous due to tumoural necrosis.

Suprarenal tumours
     Ultrasonography confirmed the presence of a mass in
9 cases,but always failed to directly assess the organ of
origin.Really this could be suspected everytime the lesion was above the kidney,dissociable from the hypocon-
driac organs (5/9 cases).
Still the large size of these tumours often did not allow
visualization of sure cleavage interfaces;at surgery,in
these cases,compression or infiltration were indifferen-
tly demonstrated.In 3 cases the tumour has been erroneously attributed to the right lobe of the liver (Fig.1).
All the tumours presented a solid highly echogenic pattern;one pheochromocytoma showed anechoic areas that,at
surgery,well correlated to massive necrosis (Fig.1).

Pancreatic tumours
     We have observed 4 pancreatic tumoural masses (2 car-
cinomas and 2 cystadenocarcinomas).Pancreatic origin
could be defined only for carcinomas;these were located
in the head of the pancreas and gave evident IVC compres-
sion.The 2 cystadenocarcinomas could not be attributed to
the pancreas.In the first case the mass was located right
to the midline:pancreatic region was obscured by bowel
gas and only CT could demonstrate that the lesion was located in the head of the pancreas and gave marked dilatation of the pancreatic duct.In the other case a large
mass was present in the left hypochondrium and diffusely
infiltrated the lower pole of the spleen.
In all these two last cases the echopattern was solid,

very inhomogeneous due both to highly reflective and a-
nechoic areas;on the contrary carcinomas presented
homogeneous echogenicity.

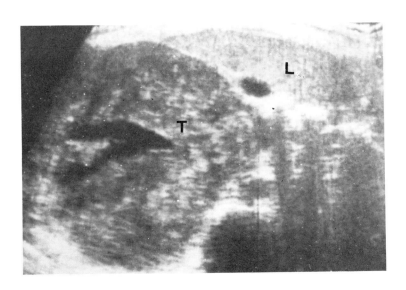

Fig.1-Anterior transverse scan through the right flank:
suprarenal pheochromocytoma(T-tumour;L-liver).

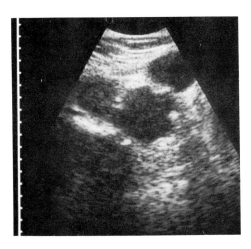

Fig.2-Anterior oblique scan through the left iliac fossa:
recurrencies of indifferentiated sarcoma.

## Retroperitoneal tumours

Seventeen tumours of the retroperitoneum presented as palpable masses.In only 11 cases we could correctly suspect the retroperitoneal origin of the lesion because this was located behind the kidney (5 cases) and the main abdominal vessels (5 cases) or tipically enclosed IVC and aorta (1 case).In the other cases the tumour either infiltrated other organs or was located anterior to the above mentioned structures and the separation between peritoneal or retroperitoneal resulted impossible. In all the 3 of these cases in which CT could be performed the visibility of the fascial planes carried out a correct diagnosis;on the other hand standard techniques were non-specific.

All the tumours showed a solid echopattern being lower reflecting than the surrounding structures;a mixed pattern with anechoic areas due to necrosis has been observed only in one case of extrarenal Wilms tumour.In 2 cases of multiple recurrencies of malignant fibrosarcoma, presenting as a single lobulated mass on physical examination,ultrasonography showed multiple low echogenic nodules;their appearance was not dissimilar to that of limphnodes involvement (Fig.2).

## DISCUSSION

In the evaluation of retroperitoneal tumours presenting as palpable masses ultrasonography shows different accuracies in relation to the requested diagnostic steps: presence of the lesion,its organ of origin,extent and nature.

## Presence of the lesion

The physical finding of a palpable mass is not always due to an effective space occupying lesion.A tortuous aorta or anteriorly displaced by an increased lumbar lordosis often simulates a pulsatile abdominal mass;in other cases renal ptosis or a vertical liver may present as a palpable mass in the right flank.In all these cases ultra sound examination is negative;quite always it explains the erroneous physical observation and no further workup is necessary.

On the other hand the effective presence of a space occupying lesion will be easily defined:the large size of these masses makes this task easier.

## Site of origin of the lesion

The recognition of the retroperitoneal origin of the mass needs that either the anatomical structure and the organ of origin or some definite anatomical landmarks are identified.

Renal origin is easily defined;even if the renal spaces are totally occupied by a total kidney tumour,the absence

of a normal kidney allows a precise diagnosis.
Suprarenal tumours are seldom correctly located.When the
mass is large enough to be detected on physical examination it is always impossible to directly define the organ of origin.Moreover compression or invasion of the
adjacent organs result in lack of cleavage interfaces (3)
and differentiation of a suprarenal lesion from a splenic
hepatic or an upper-pole renal mass is therefore difficult.
Some doubts may exist also for pancreatic tumours.Only
cystadenocarcinomas often reveal as palpable masses (5);
neoplastic symptoms,jaundice and secondary liver involvement are in fact the most frequent presenting findings
for pancreatic carcinoma.When a mass is present still ultrasonography may fail correct location due both to the
large size of the tumour and the absence of anatomical
landmarks (5).
As it concerns the primary tumours of the retroperitoneum
they grow much in size and displace or often infiltrate
the adjacent structures;when liver or spleen are deeply
involved they may be erroneously considered as the site
of origin (1).
In some of those cases in which ultrasonography fails to
define a precise anatomical structure or an organ of origin,the mass can however be correctly located in the retroperitoneal space;this happens everytime the mass is
behind kidneys,pancreas,liver,spleen,aorta,IVC or mesenteric vessels.On the contrary the retroperitoneal or peritoneal origin can not be defined for masses located
anterior to the kidneys;in fact,due to the absence of interfaces,ultrasonography do not allow visualization of
the posterior parietal peritoneum and of the anterior renal fascia (1).
Coupling ultrasound to other imaging modalities (IVP,ba-
rium studies,etc.) certainly makes correct location easier;nevertheless CT,allowing both to easily recognize
some anatomical structures (suprarenal glands,pancreas,u-
reters and opacified bowel loops) and to localize the lesion in relation to the fascial compartments,is clearly
superior to ultrasonography (11).

Extent of the lesion
     Several reports have pointed out the possibilities of
ultrasonography in the evaluation of the tumoural extent
as it regards both limphnodes and vessels involvement
(3,11).As for retroperitoneal masses we believe that sufficient accuracy may be achieved only for tumours originating in the upper right retroperitoneum,right renal tumours being quite well staged with regards to renal vein
or IVC thrombosis;nevertheless fascial infiltration or
small suprarenal metastases,quite easily detected by CT,
escape diagnosis.Worse informations are obtained for tumours located in the lower retroperitoneum.Limitations

are strictly linked to the physical nature of ultrasound;
bony structures and bowel gas often prevent good visualization of the mass and,even if this is large enough to
displace the intestines,the peripheral extentions of the
tumour are difficult to define.Ureteral involvement can
be indirectly suspected when hydronephrosis is present
but we absolutely need to further perform an IVP to determine the degree and the extent of either compression
or infiltration;moreover ultrasonography gives no information about fatty or bony structures invasion and the
fascial planes can not be defined.
Some of the above mentioned limitations may be only partially overcome by using appropriate scanning techniques
(10) and well focussed transducers;yet high-resolution
dynamic scanners,mechanical sectors in particular,seem to
be promising.

Nature of the lesion
     With a very few exceptions the retroperitoneal tu-
mours appear as solid masses.Echogenicity may be different varying from highly reflective lesions to ipoechoic
or very inhomogeneous masses.Previous reports tried to
correlate these echopatterns to the vascularity (9) or
to the fatty or fibrous content (2,4,8) of the lesion.
Our experience confirms that every attempt to get specific correlations gives disappointing results.Moreover
benign and malignant tumours may present similar patterns,
inflammatory lesions may mimic neoplasms and multiple recurrencies may simulate limphnodes involvement.Therefore
the identification of a solid mass allows only a presumptive diagnosis of neoplasm;ultrasonically guided biopsy
could certainly give good pathological specimens and
laparoscopy would be no more necessary.It must also be
stressed that not all the retroperitoneal malignant tumours have a solid echopattern;in fact it has been well
demonstrated that either for their pathologic characteristics (5) or for extensive necrosis (12) some retroperitoneal neoplasms may present as anechoic masses.

CONCLUSIONS

     Finding a mass on physical examination requires to
the physician to confirm the presence of an effective lesion and to achieve more definite informations about its
organ of origin,extent and nature.
     Ultrasonography is now so widely diffuse that in the-
se cases is very often requested as first examination
instead of other diagnostic techniques commonly used in
the past.
Facing with the problem of the effective presence of a
lesion the diagnostic impact of ultrasonography is impressive;on the other hand,failing the preliminary informations that previously used imaging methods could sup-

ply,ultrasound alone reveal some limitations when used to evaluate retroperitoneal tumours.Ultrasonography seems particularly limited in locating the lesion in relation to its organ of origin and to the fascial compartments and in determining the actual tumoural extent;moreover the differential diagnosis with other benign masses is often difficult.
Nevertheless a diagnostic approach based on plain film and ultrasonography as initial procedures is effective; in fact in quite all the cases an ultrasound examination coupled with an IVP or a barium enema provides sufficient information prior to surgery.But considering an up-to-da te oncological treatment CT still seems to be the imaging procedure of choice.

REFERENCES

1. Bazzocchi,M.,Maffessanti,M.,Pozzi-Mucelli,R.S. et Al. (1980):In:Atti V Congresso Nazionale SISUM,p.51.Editors:De Albertis,P. and Colagrande,C.Novappia,Roma
2. Behan,M. and Kazam,E.(1978):Radiology,129,143
3. Bernardino,M.E.,Goldstein,H.M. and Green,B.(1978): AJR,130,741
4. Bree,R.L. and Green,B.(1978):Radiology,128,193
5. Busilacchi,P.,Rizzatto,G.,Bazzocchi,M. et Al.(1982): Br.J.Radiol.,in press.
6. Duncan,R.E. and Evans,A.(1977):J.Urol.,117,19
7. Goldstein,H.M.,Green,B. and Weaver,R.M.(1978):AJR, 130,1083
8. Kurtz,A.B.,Dubbins,P.A.,Rubin,C.S. et Al.(1981):AJR, 137,471
9. Makland,N.F.,Chuang,V.P.,Doust,B.B. et Al.(1977): Radiology,123,733
10. Sample,W.F.(1977):Radiology,124,197
11. Whalen,J.P.(1979):AJR,133,585
12. Yeh,H.,Mitty,H.A.,Rose,J. et Al.(1978):Radiology, 127,475

# ECHOGRAPHIC FINDINGS IN CARCINOMA OF RENAL PELVIS

Massimo Bazzocchi, Giorgio Rizzatto, Roberto S. PozziMucelli, Claudio Ricci and Ludovico DallaPalma

*Institute of Radiology, Ospedale Maggiore, University of Trieste, Trieste, Italy*

Renal pelvis tumours (RPT) are usually transitional cell tumours and rapresent 5-10% of renal neoplasms(2,4).

The diagnosis of RPT is based on urography in most of cases(1,3).

The retrograde pyelography and arteriography may give some diagnostic informations(5).

The radiological diagnosis may be uncertain in case of a urographic doubtful filling defect,or in case of a non functioning kidney.

Recently ultrasounds (U.S.) have been proposed for the evaluation of the RPT,and of the renal pelvis radio lucent stones(6,7,8).

U.S. were performed in a group of patients for the evaluation of RPT: the results are reported.

MATERIALS AND METHODS

Has been evaluated 19 patients with monolateral RPT; the ureter was involved in 3 cases, while a tumour of the bladder was present in 2 other cases.

All patients underwent urography and U.S..The exa minations has been performed with available dinamic and static scanners( with 3.5 MHz transducers ).

RESULTS

Three different patterns were observed in our series
1) no modifications of the normal echogenicity of the si nus was noted in 5 cases; the sinus was normal in 3 cases,while hydronephrosis was the only finding in 2 other cases. In 3 cases small multiple neoplastic loca lizations were present: urography correctly showed these cases. In 2 out of 5 cases urography showed a single filling defect.

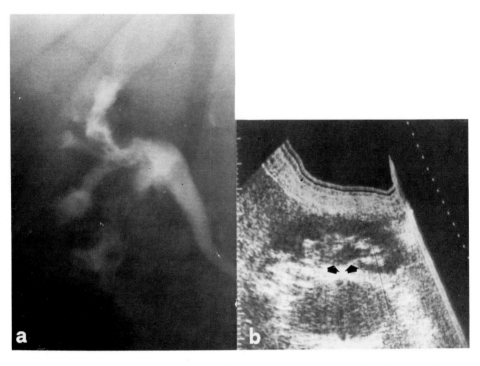

Figure 1. RPT: in urography(a) many pelvic filling defects in U.S.(b),longitudinal scan,ipoechoic mass in the sinus reproducing caliceal morphology.

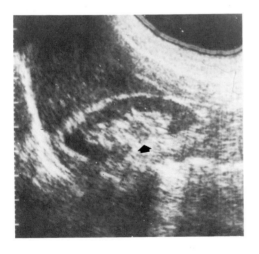

Figure 2. RPT: longitudi‐ nal scan.Sinusal mass well separated from the inner contour of the renal pa‐ renchima.

2) a sinusal mass was seen in 13 cases. The echogenicity
   of the mass wass the same of the renal parenchima in
   11 cases,while was hyperechoic in 2 cases,less echoic
   however than the sinus.
   The tumoural mass was completely or almost separated
   from the inner contour of therenal parenchima.
   This finding enabled us to suspect the origin from the
   renal pelvis. At urography the origin from the renal
   pelvis was suspected in 10 cases: in 2 cases urography
   showed a non functioning kidney and in 1 case the uro
   graphic aspect of the lesion was consistent with a
   parenchimal tumour.
   The morphology of the mass was similar to the dilated
   renal pelvis and calices in 9 cases (Fig. 1).
   In these cases the mass was separated in all its
   extension from the inner contour of the renal paren
   chima (Fig. 2); histological examination confirmed
   the ultrasonographic findings,that the mass was confi
   ned inside the sinus.
   No defined morphology was recognized in 4 cases. In
   these cases the mass was not completely demarcated
   inside the sinus. Hystology confirmed the parenchimal
   infiltration only in 1 case.
   In no cases the extension of the lesion could be defi
   ned by urography.

3) U.S. showed a large solid mass in 1 case of non
   functioning kidney at urography.
   This was a large RPT which obstructed the pelvis and
   caused hydropionephrosis. The debris caused the solid
   pattern at U.S..

CONCLUSIONS

In evaluating RPT,U.S. may give either no findings
or a not specific aspect of a sinusal mass.
However U.S. is complementary to urography because
it may add diagnostic informations in some situations:
in the definition of a non functioning kidney,in the
definition of the nature of the lesion particularly in
the differential diagnosis with radiolucent stones, in
the diagnosis of origin of the lesion from the pelvis,
and finally in the evaluation of the sinusal extension
of an intraluminal tumours.

# REFERENCES

1. Geerdsen,J.,(1979) Scand.J.Urol.Nephrol13,287.
2. Grace,D.A.,Taylor,W.N.,Taylor,J.N.,Winter,C.C.(1967)
   J.Urol. 87,566.
3. Leong,C.H.,Lim,T.K.,Wong,K.K.,Ong,G.B.(1976): Br.J.
   Surg. 63,102.
4. Melen,D.R.(1944): J.Urol. 51,386.
5. Michel,J.R.,Vital,J.L.,Moreau,J.F.,Affre,J. (1975):
   J.Radiol.Electrol. 56,875.
6. Mulholland,S.G.,Arger,P.H.,Goldberg,B.B.,Pollack,H.M.
   (1979): J.Urol. 122,14
7. Rosenfield,A.T.,Taylor,K.J.W.,Dembner,A.G.,Jacobson,P.
   (1979): A.J.R. 133,441.

# DIAGNOSIS OF PROSTATIC CANCER WITH TRANSRECTAL ULTRASONOTOMOGRAPHY

Hiroki Watanabe

*Department of Urology, Kyoto Prefectural University of Medicine, Kyoto, Japan 602*

## INTRODUCTION

The prostate is a male accessory sexual organ which is located just beneath the urinary bladder, surrounding the urethra. It is normally the size of a walnut. It lies in front of the rectum, and can therefore be palpated easily by digital examination.

From this anatomical structure, two important diseases of the prostate, benign prostatic hypertrophy and prostatic cancer, which result in prostatic enlargement, both show a similar symptom --- dysuria.

Benign prostatic hypertrophy is not a malignant tumor but an adenomatous hyperplasia. It is one of the most prevalent diseases among the senile male population of any country. Prostatic cancer is malignant and is the second or third most prevalent cancer in males in American and European countries. Accordingly, both diseases are significantly important in geriatric medicine.

For over two thousand years, digital palpation has been almost the only way to examine the prostate. However, for diagnostic purposes palpation is too dependent upon the physician's skill and experience. Several types of x-ray studies are also of some value as diagnostic means but they can only indirectly procure representation of the prostatic space.

## TRANSRECTAL ULTRASONOTOMOGRAPHY

Transrectal ultrasonotomography is a new diagnostic technique whereby this blind spot in the prostatic examination can be eliminated. With this technique the anatomic structure of the prostate is visible in the form of an easily comprehensible cross-section map.[1]

The actual procedure is carried out with the patient sitting in the examination chair,[2,3] the seat of which is covered with a disposable rubber mat. A special probe, 12 mm in diameter, is smoothly inserted into the rectum by rotating a handle beneath the chair. The tip of the probe is wrapped in a specially designed disposable rubber balloon, which can be attached or detached instantly (Fig. 1).

The balloon is filled with water to maintain contact

Table 1. Diagnostic criteria in transrectal ultrasonotomography for the prostate (Watanabe)

| Findings \ Diseases | Normal | Hypertrophy | Cancer | Prostatitis |
|---|---|---|---|---|
| Shape of section | Triangular or semilunar | Enlarged Nearly round | Irregular Deformed | Enlarged in acute cases Deformed in chronic cases |
| Anteroposterior diameter | Short | Elongated | Elongated but with some exceptions | Usually short |
| Superoinferior diameter | Short | Elongated, associated with anteroposterior diameter | Occasionally elongated and unbalanced | Usually short |
| Symmetry | Present | Present | Absent | Absent |
| Change of shape on each level | Little | Little | Marked | Little |
| Capsular echoes { Thickness | Thin | Thick | Irregular | Irregular if invaded |
| Continuity | Present | Present | Absent | Usually present |
| Unevenness | Absent | Absent | Present | Present |
| Internal echoes { Density | (+) | (++) | (+) | (++) in chronic cases |
| Quality | Orderly | Orderly | Disorderly but occasionally disappears | Disorderly |

with the rectal wall. Radial scanning is performed automatically. No treatment is necessary prior to the examination, and the entire procedure requires only several minutes.

In our recent evaluation of the function of the equipment in our clinic in Kyoto Prefectural University of Medicine during the approximately 3 years from June, 1976 to February, 1980, the examination was performed 3,000 times on 2,331 patients[4]. The examination was unsuccessful only 21 times (0.7%). The causes of failure were as follows: incomplete insertion of the probe in 5 cases, minor hypotensive episodes in 4 cases, rupture of the balloon in 4 cases, insufficient bladder expantion in 1 case, and malfunction of the camera in 7 cases. No particular complication was observed in this series.

Thus the functioning of the equipment seems to be excellent. The occurrence of failures or complications was thought to be negligibly small.

In the diagnosis of prostatic diseases, three major findings should be noticed. They are the deformity of the prostatic section, the change of the capsular echoes which are the linear echo patterns caused by the prostatic capsule, and also the change of the internal echoes which are the echo patterns distributed inside the prostate caused by the prostatic substance (Table 1).

The horizontal tomogram of the prostate in normal subjects is usually obtained when the probe is inserted to a depth of several cms from the anus. The normal prostate is seen as a slender triangular or semilunar pattern (Fig. 2, upper left).

In patients with acute prostatitis, a diffuse swelling of the prostatic shape and a decrease in the number of internal echoes are usually observed.

In patients with chronic prostatitis, various kinds of prostatic deformity showing irregularity on the capsular echoes and the internal echoes can be observed in various degrees according to the stage of the disease (Fig. 2, upper right).

The section of the prostate in patients with benign prostatic hypertrophy is enlarged symmetrically, most noticeable along the A-P diameter. The shape of the prostatic section is semilunar in the early stages and is nearly round or oval in the advanced stages (Fig. 2, below left).

DIAGNOSIS OF PROSTATIC CANCER

The characteristic finding of the prostate involved in cancer can be summarized in one word --- irregularity. There is no prostatic disease other than cancer which shows such a variety of pattern on the section.

The shapes of prostatic sections show deformity and asymmetry from the early stages. Though the enlargement of the prostatic section occurs with a balance between the

Table 2. Differentiation between cancer
         and chronic prostatitis

|  | Cancer | Chronic prostatitis |
|---|---|---|
| Size | Large | Medium |
| Symmetry | Highly asymmetric | Relatively symmetric |
| Shape on different levels | Non-analogous | Analogous |

Table 3. Ultrasonic and final diagnosis
         in prostatic cancer

| Ultrasonic diagnosis | Prostatic cancer | Suspected prostatic cancer | Other prostatic diseases |
|---|---|---|---|
| Final diagnosis | | | |
| Prostatic cancer (+) | 54 (94.7%) | 12 ( 3.7%) | 2 ( 0.1%) |
| Prostatic cancer (−) | 3 ( 5.3%) | 314 (96.3%) | 1,739 (99.9%) |
| Total | 57 | 326 | 1,741 |

Table 4. Result of mass screening
         (Jan., 1975–June, 1981)

| Examinee | 612 |
|---|---|
| Average age | 62.9 y.o. |
| Cases for secondary study | 276 (45.1%) |
| Final diagnosis | |
| BPH Stage I | 155 (25.3%) |
| BPH Stage II | 40 ( 6.5%) |
| Prostatic cancer | 6 ( 1.0%) |
| Prostatitis | 20 ( 3.3%) |
| Miscellaneous | 12 ( 2.0%) |

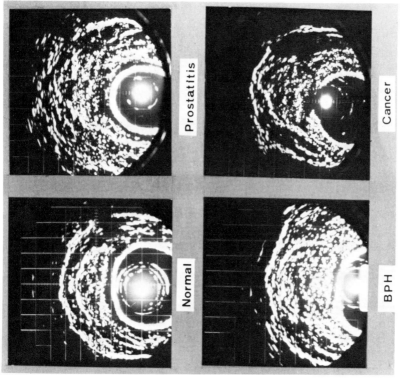

Fig. 2. Horizontal section of the prostate in verious prostatic diseases.

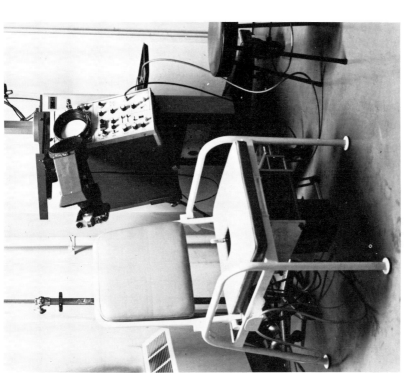

Fig. 1. Chair-type equipment for trans-rectal ultrasonotomography.

251

A-P and the lateral diameter in cases of benign prostatic hypertrophy, in cancer cases it is often unbalanced. The capsular echoes are still continuous when no infiltration has occurred but their thickness is uneven. The internal echoes are also irregular. In some instances in the early stages, the number of internal echoes decreases so that the overall inside region shows as a dark area (Fig. 3).

In advanced cases, the deformity and asymmetry are more pronounced. A special elongation on the A-P diameter is often remarkable. Both the capsular and the internal echoes become highly irregular. The prostatic shapes on different levels are not analogous to each other. Infiltration of surrounding tissues by cancer can be seen as a protrusion of prostatic substance with a discontinuity of the capsular echoes (Fig. 2, below right).

For the diagnosis of prostatic cancer, it is extremely important to examine all the sections carefully because difference of the prostatic shape on each tomogram taken at different levels is a particular finding in cancer. On the contrary, in cases of benign prostatic hypertrophy, the prostatic shape is always similar.

Changes of prostatic section in hypertrophy and cancer are demonstrated schematically on Fig. 4. In a normal subject, the prostate is seen as a slender triangular or semilunar pattern, with the A-P diameter shorter than the bilateral diameter. The section in benign prostatic hypertrophy enlarges equally in peripheral directions, approaching a thick semilunar pattern in early cases and a circular pattern in advanced cases. On the contrary, the section in cancer occasionally has a special elongation on the A-P diameter out of balance with the bilateral diameter and resulting in a "bell" shape.[5]

This can be seen from Fig. 5 which shows a section of advanced prostatic cancer. A mild extracapsular infiltration is suspected from a discontinuity of the capsular echoes.

As already mentiond, the A-P diameter of the prostatic section is elongated in usual cancer cases. Although it is rather rare, an elongation only on the bilateral diameter can sometimes be found, as shown on Fig. 6.

In my early papers[1,2,3] I described that it was difficult to differentiate between cancer and chronic inflammation by this method. But over the last several years, having had experience of more than 2,000 cases, I have begun to change my opinion. At present in our clinic differentiation is in fact usually possible. The secret is very simple --- to keep firmly to the diagnostic criteria I proposed. One should notice the three points shown on Table 2.

STAGING OF PROSTATIC CANCER

According to the classification of the staging of prostatic cancer on the American system, Stage A means

Normal: triangular or
semilunar

BPH: thick semilunar or
circular

Cancer: "bell" shape

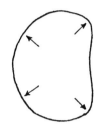

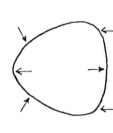

Fig. 4. Schematic demonstration of
changes of prostatic section.

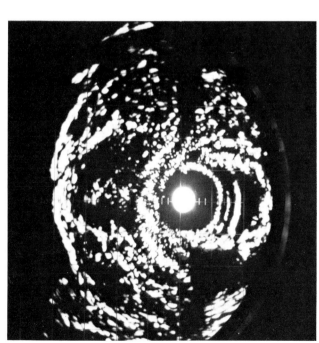

Fig. 3. Early prostatic cancer.

that the cancer is completely restricted within the prostate including latent cancer, Stage B that the cancer involves almost the whole prostate without extracapsular infiltration, Stage C that the cancer is beyond the capsule, and Stage D that a distant metastasis is evident.

Whether Stage A cancer can be detected by transrectal ultrasonotomography or not is a very interesting question. In our clinic we have encountered only one case of Stage A cancer. We failed to diagnose this as cancer. It might be theoretically impossible to find a tiny cancer focus a few mm in diameter by ultrasound.

For this reason, whether differentiation between Stage A and B by this method is possible or not is not clear. However, from our experience, cancer cells were always proved in any portion of the specimen of the resected prostate which had shown deformity on the tomogram prior to surgery. We presume, accordingly, that when deformity has been observed on the tomogram of the prostate in early prostatic cancer, the case might be considered to be Stage B.

Transrectal ultrasonotomography is very useful for differentiation between Stages B and C. As mentioned above, differentiation is achieved by evaluating the condition of the capsular echoes. Not only the existence of infiltration but its location and degree can easily be described. The advantage of this method is augmented by the fact that there is a very distinct difference in the treatment and prognosis of prostatic cancer which are under Stage B and over Stage C.

The staging of prostatic cancer has until now only been made by palpation. However, in many cases ultrasound detected clear infiltration which could not be revealed by palpation.

Stage D is confirmed mainly by roentgenography or scintigraphy. For this purpose, transrectal ultrasonotomography is useful only in cases with infiltration into surrounding organs, such as the bladder or the seminal vesicles.

DIAGNOSTIC ACCURACY IN PROSTATIC CANCER

To confirm the diagnostic accuracy of transrectal ultrasonotomography in prostatic cancer, we made an evaluation of the previously mentioned 3,000 cases which had undergone the examination in our clinic in Kyoto from June, 1976 to February, 1980[4]

In 57 patients diagnosed as having prostatic cancer by transrectal ultrasonotomography, 54 (94.7%) were finally diagnosed as having cancer by biopsy. In 326 patients who were suspected of prostatic cancer by ultrasound, 12 (3.7%) were also confirmed as having cancer by biopsy. However, among 1,741 patients with various prostatic diseases on whom cancer was ruled out by ultrasound, we found only 2 (0.1%) false-negative cases with cancer (Table 3).

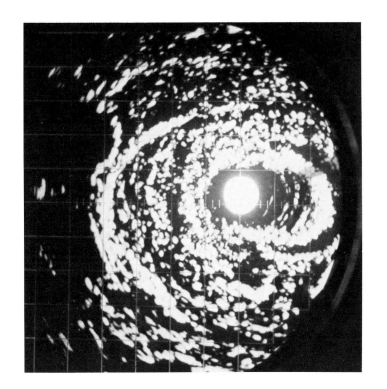

Fig. 6. Advanced prostatic cancer with an elongation of lateral diameter.

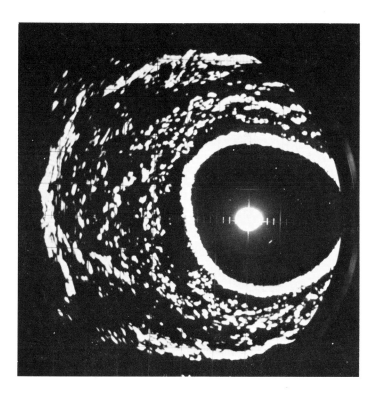

Fig. 5. Advanced prostatic cancer in "bell" shape.

SIZE MEASUREMENT OF THE PROSTATE

It is well known that ultrasonic techniques are able to make precise measurements of the sizes of various organs. In urology it is of practical importance to measure the size and weight of the prostate[6].

By means of transrectal ultrasonotomography, tomograms can be recorded routinely every 5 mm of depth of insertion of the transducer into the rectum, on 35 mm black and white film.

The prostatic weight is estimated as the sum of the area of each section. The area of prostatic section on each tomogram taken at 5 mm intervals is measured by a roller planimeter. The area of section multiplied by 0.5 can be taken to be the volume of a section of the prostate 0.5 cm in thickness. This prostatic volume can be taken to be approximately equal to the prostatic weight, because the specific gravity of prostatic tissue is about 1.0 according to our measurements of surgically excised specimens.

Twenty-four cases of prostatic cancer without any prior treatment were treated only by castration, and the volume of the prostate was measured ultrasonically before and after castration very frequently. Measurement was taken almost every day in the first postoperative week and every two days in the second postoperative week. After the third postoperative week it was taken once or twice per week.

Fig. 7 shows the regression curves of the prostatic volume in these cases. It seems that the volume reduced exponentially in each case after therapy, approaching a constant plateau level without exception. There is a possibility that a kinetic analysis like this will open a new aspect to cancer therapeutics.

MASS SCREENING PROGRAM FOR PROSTATIC DISEASES

Transrectal ultrasonotomography is suitable as a screening test for prostatic diseases. We originated a system for a mass screening program for this purpose using the technique as the primary study[7]. It revealed an astonishingly high prevalence of benign prostatic hypertrophy and prostatic cancer in apparently normal older males.

We developed a mobile unit for the mass screening of prostatic diseases in December, 1980[8] (Fig. 8). It has two sets of special equipment for transrectal ultrasonotomography and a recording system in the cabin. While one examinee is being examined on one chair, the next examinee is requested to prepare himself on another chair. The average time required per person is 3.3 minutes including preparation and wasted time. The primary study on over one-hundred persons can be performed in one day.

We have carried out the mass screening on 612 male

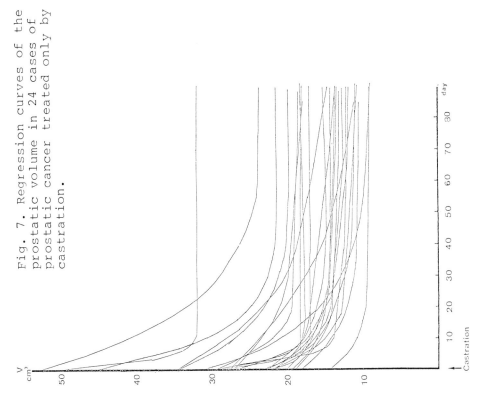

Fig. 7. Regression curves of the prostatic volume in 24 cases of prostatic cancer treated only by castration.

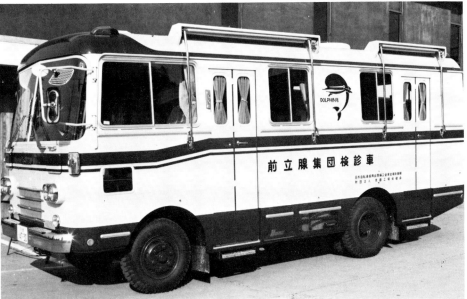

Fig. 8. Mobile unit for the mass screening of prostatic diseases.

subjects more than 55 years of age by this system up until June, 1981. Benign prostatic hypertrophy was detected in approximately 30% and prostatic cancer in approximately 1% of them (Table 4). It was thus proved that the system is both reliable and efficient.

CONCLUSION

In my first paper on transrectal ultrasonotomography in 1971[1], I made the prediction that "this procedure will become one of the most important means of examination for diagnosing prostatic diseases in the near future". Now, ten years afterwards, this is being realized. In Japan, many major hospitals have adopted the technique as the most reliable diagnostic means for investigating the prostate. Several different types of scanners for the same use are now being distributed by a number of makers throughout the World. I hope the technique will come to be used in most urological clinics over the next ten years.

REFERENCES

1. Watanabe, H., et al. (1971): Invest. Urol., 8, 548.
2. Watanabe, H., et al. (1974): J. Clin. Ultrasound, 2 91.
3. Watanabe, H., et al. (1975): J. Urol., 114, 734.
4. Watanabe, H., et al. (1980): The Prostate, 1, 271.
5. Watanabe, H. (1981): In: Diagnostic Ultrasound in Urology and Nephrology, p.130.
   Editors: Hiroki Watanabe et al. Igaku-Shoin, Tokyo.
6. Watanabe, H., et al. (1974): Tohoku J. Exp. Med., 114, 277.
7. Watanabe, H., et al. (1977): J. Urol., 117, 746.
8. Ohe, H., et al. (1981): Med. Technol., 9, 873. (Jap.)

# BLADDER CANCER STAGING BY TRANSURETHRAL ULTRASONOGRAPHY

L. Denis, J. Braeckman and M. Chaban

*Departments of Urology, A.Z. VUB Brussels and A.Z. Middelheim, Antwerp, Belgium*

Major improvements in ultrasound imaging technology have greatly increased the clinical value of ultrasonography in lower urinary tract pathology (1,2). The ultrasonography of the bladder can be performed by three different techniques: the transabdominal scan, the transrectal radial scan and the transurethral radial scan (3).

This report summarizes our clinical experience with the transurethral scan in the staging of bladder cancer. The first transurethral radial scanner was developed in the laboratory of Holm (4). The principle of the real time transurethral scanner utilized in this study was first described by Nakamura (5).

## PRINCIPLE

Short bursts of alternating electrical current generate sonic energy in a piezoelectric crystal. This sonic energy, usually at a frequency from 2 to 7.5 megahertz, is emmitted in sound waves that form a beam. Whenever these sound waves strike tissue with different acoutstic properties part of the sonic energy is reflected. These returning echoes are captured by the crystal and through conversion reproduced as position specific echo dots forming a bidimensional cross-section of the examined structures. A sequence of cross-sections allows a tomographic reconstruction. The acoustic difference of a tissue depends on the acoustic impedance, acoustic impedance being the product of the density of a substance and the velocity of sound in that particular substance. The greater the difference in acoustic impedance the higher the amplitude of the returned echoes. The reflecting echoes produced by the bladder are of two kinds. The high amplitude echoes or specular reflections generated by the wall of the bladder and the low amplitude echoes or diffuse reflections generated by tissue material in the water filled bladder with less acoustic impedance as mucosal hypertrophy, blood clots but most important bladder tumors (Figs. 1, 2).

## EQUIPMENT

The combination transabdominal, transrectal and transurethral scanning equipment (Aloka SSD 501) consists of a multi-purpose imaging unit and interchangable scanners. The pulsed echo dots are displayed as transsectional images in a real time viewing system. This high speed viewing system increases efficiency and patient throughput time. The image on the oscilloscope is provided with date and identification markers and caliper dot markers.

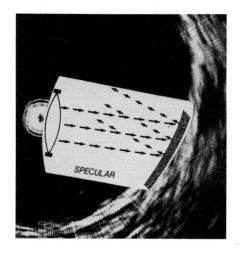
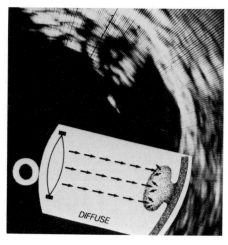

Fig.1 Ultrasound waves hitting
the bladder wall generate high
amplitude or specular reflections. Sharpest contrast is obtained by a perpendicular hit
(left).

Fig.2 Diffuse reflections represent the form and consistency of
intraluminal structures in the
bladder. Note the sessile bladder
tumor in the dome of the bladder
(right).

The radial urethral scanner is pistol shaped. Two crystals with
a diameter of 0.5 cm of a 7.5 megahertz focus type are fixed to a
transducer. One crystal located at 1.5 cm from the top is fixed
in a 90° angle. A similar crystal is fixed one cm. lower in a 120°
angle. This lower crystal allows a perpendicular sonic beam to be
utilized in screening tumors located near the bladder neck (Fig. 3).
The transducer probe system fits into a 24 Charriere sheath and
protrudes out of the sheath in the bladder. The scanning speed can
be adjusted from 10 rotations per second. Serial pictures are taken
from the screen by video-recording or specially adapted Polaroid
photography. The scanner can be attached to a scanner stand which
can be moved in 1 mm intervals parallel to the long axis of the
probe.

PROCEDURE

Transurethral ultrasound scanning is performed as an integral part
of the diagnostic cystoscopic work up in bladder cancer which
includes visual description of abnormalities present, introduction
of the transurethral scanner followed by the scanning procedure,
introduction of the resectoscope sheath followed by biopsies of
normal looking mucosa by cold cup biopsy forceps and finished by a
resection and fulguration of the visible tumor (6). The diagnostic
work up is performed on a patient under general anesthesia in the
usual lithotomy position. The total scanning procedure takes five
to ten minutes. The bladder is filled without overstretching after
introduction of the transurethral scanner. The filling of the bladder

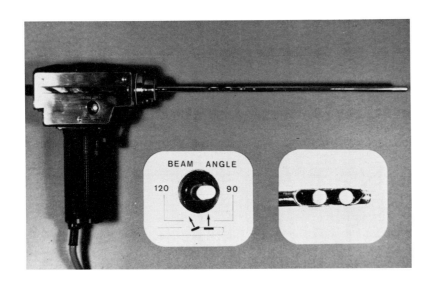

Fig.3 Model of the transurethral radial scanner. The difference in beam angle allows a perpendicular scanning independent of the location of the tumor in the bladder.

is easy to follow on the screen. The transducer is represented by a circle in the bladder. The air bubble is strongly echogenic and forms a constant landmark. The ureters are visualized especially when dilated.

After the location of the air bubble, we start our scanning from the dome to the bladder neck in sequential steps usually at 0.5 cm. Representative photographs are taken in a routine procedure (Fig. 4).

RESULTS

The transurethral scanning was performed on 72 patients scheduled for cystoscopy and random biopsy procedures. In 72 patients tumor mass was present and the sonographic staging was compared to the T staging after transurethral resection (7) according to the TNM classification of malignant tumors (8) (Table 1).

Table 1. Correlation between T staging by transurethral resection and transurethral preoperative ultrasound.

| TUR | $T_1$ | $T_2$ | $T_3$ | TOTAL |
|---|---|---|---|---|
| Ultrasound | | | | |
| $T_1$ | 57 | 2 | 0 | 59 |
| $T_2$ | 0 | 7 | 0 | 7 |
| $T_3$ | 0 | 0 | 6 | 6 |
| TOTAL | 57 | 9 | 6 | 72 |

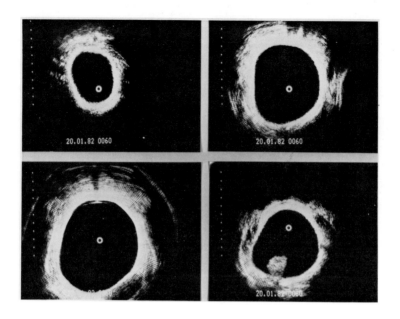

Fig.4 Sequential sonograms of the bladder filled with 200 cc of
saline. Starting from the dome top left, a transsection 1 cm lower
top right, still lower a transsection through the body of the bladder
with the air bubble at the top lower left and the final section with
a solitary T1 tumor clearly visible. Note the position of the transducer in every picture.

    The normal bladder appears as a symmetrical, smooth gently cur-
ved surface.  The bladder wall is an even, continuous echogenic structure of oval or round shape depending on the degree of distension.
Defects caused by dilated submucosal ureters or diverticulae are
easily recognized.
    Normal bladder mucosa can not be distinguished from the muscular
layers of the bladder wall.  Ghost echoes originating from tiny air
bubbles or loose material inside the bladder are easily recognized
as artifacts by a different positioning of the transducer.
    Hypertrophy of the mucosa is visualized as an echo poor layer
on the bladder wall.  A tissue mass fixed to the bladder wall is
easily recognized.as a bladder cancer.  In a proper plane the tumor
can already be visualized through a transabdominal or a transrectal
scan but a transurethral scan is essential for accurate determination
of tumor infiltration (Fig. 5).
    The perpendicular scan ascertains the infiltration of the
bladder wall as in T2 bladder tumors (Fig. 6 top).
    Papillary tumors present by their diffuse echoes as spongy
masses while solid tumors are less echogenic as represented in this
T3b tumor with a complete penetration of the bladder wall (Fig. 6).

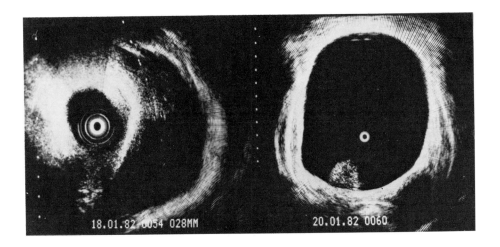

Fig.5 This solitary sessile bladder tumor was already detected by transrectal ultrasonography during an observation for prostatic pathology (left). The transurethral sonogram shows a sessile tumor on an intact bladder wall (right).

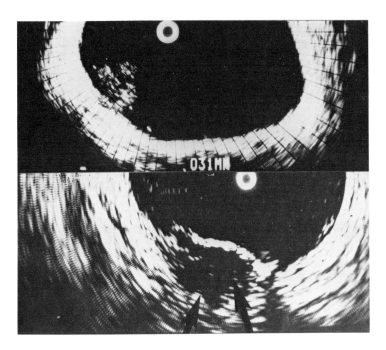

Fig.6 The infiltration of this T2 tumor is clearly visible by the defect in the bladder wall (top). Total penetration by a T3b solid tumor is obvious (below).

Tumor surface and mass inside the bladder are easily evaluated by the dot caliper markers and tomographic reconstruction in sequential steps (Fig. 7).

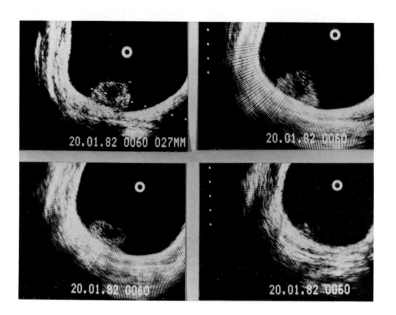

Fig.7 Tomographic mass reconstruction of a bladder tumor is possible by dot markers and sequential sonograms. In this example taken every 3 mm.

DISCUSSION

After five years of experience with transabdominal and transrectal ultrasonic techniques (3) we prefer transurethral ultrasonography for the staging of bladder tumors. It is however important to emphasize that ultrasonography can not be seen as an isolated technique and should be evaluated as to its proper place in staging bladder cancer in conjunction with established diagnostic modalities.
    The proper place is the differential diagnosis between Ta/T1 and T2/T3 tumors. The differential diagnosis between Ta and T1 tumors is impossible for it exceeds the limitations of the technique. The differential diagnosis between T2 and T3 tumors depends on the clear detail of the bladder wall under the tumor. This differentiation is possible with the perpendicular approach to screen infiltration. Microscopic infiltration as in one of our cases is of course impossible to detect. False positive reports - overstaging - have been reported by Niijima (9) when unsuspected calcifications are present in the tumor.
    We do not utilize this technique for screening of bladder tumors. On many occassions bladder tumors are detected by transabdominal or transrectal ultrasonography. We utilize these techniques in our routine work up for prostatic problems since both techniques are non invasive and completely painless. We used the transurethral

technique to check on the location of multiple tumors but the new fish eye cystoscopic lenses have outgrown this time consuming procedure.

Once the tumor has infiltrated into the pelvis it is impossible to evaluate these T4 tumors since their size excludes measurement by the limited range and focus of the transducer. Mass determination in voluminous or grossly infiltrating tumors and the relation to the other pelvic organs should be done by computerized tomography (10).

We belive that the possiblity of preoperative staging is of clinical benefit to the patient whenlocal radiation treatment in superficial bladder tumors awaits to be applied in our clinical praxis.

REFERENCES

1. Resnick, M. and Sanders, R.C. (1979): Ultrasound in Urology. The Williams and Wilkins Company, Baltimore.

2. Watanabe, H., Holmes, J.H., Holm, H.H. and Goldberg, B.B. (1981): Diagnostic Ultrasound in Urology and Nephrology, Tokyo, Igahu-Shoin.

3. Denis, L. (1981): Evaluation of Lower Urinary Tract Pathology by Ultrasonography in Advances in Diagnostic Urology, p. 146. Editor: C. Schulman. Springer-Verlag, Berlin.

4. Holm, H.H. and Northeved, A. (1974): A transurethral ultrasonic scanner. J. Urol., III, 238.

5. Nakamura, S. and Niijima, T. (1981): Transurethral real-time scanner. J. Urol., 125, 781.

6. Prout, G.R. Jr (1982): Dynamic Evaluation of Bladder Cancer in Clinical Bladder Cancer, p. 61. Editors: L. Denis, P.H. Smith and M. Pavone-Macaluso. Plenum Press, New York.

7. Pavone-Macaluso, M. (1982): Staging of Bladder Cancer in Clinical Bladder Cancer, p. 37. Editors: L. Denis, P.H. Smith and M. Pavone-Macaluso. Plenum Press, New York.

8. U.I.C.C. (1978): TNM Classification of Malignant Tumors, Geneva.

9. Niijima, T. and Nakamura, S. (1982): Transurethral Ultrasonography: Bladder Cancer staging and other clinical applications in Clinical Bladder Cancer, p. 47. Editors: L. Denis, P.H. Smith and M. Pavone-Macaluso. Plenum Press, New York.

10. Declercq, G., Denis, L., Broos, J. and Appel, L. (1981): Evaluation of Lower Urinary Tract by Computed Tomography and Transrectal Ultrasonography. Comp. Tom., 5, 153.

# ULTRASONIC EVALUATION AND FOLLOW-UP IN PEDIATRIC ABDOMINAL ONCOLOGY

M. Spehl, C. Bogaert, C. Christophe, J. Otten[1] and N. Perlmutter-Cremer

*Department of Pediatric Radiology and [1]Department of Pediatrics, Hôpital Universitaire St. Pierre, ULB-VUB, University of Brussels, Brussels, Belgium*

## INTRODUCTION

Abdominal echography has become widely used in pediatrics as a diagnostic tool in every day practice.
It is a non invasive and painless investigation that can be repeated as often as necessary.
Abdominal grey scale or real time examination can be used to advantage in the evaluation and follow up of children with neoplastic diseases by helping to detect the malignant process, to evaluate its extent, to detect metastasis, and by following its response to treatment. It is also a good follow up screening test to detect a relapse.
The purpose of this paper is to illustrate the usefulness of ultrasound in the diagnosis and follow up of the course of neoplastic disease in small children.

## TECHNIQUE

B mode digital grey scale and real time sector scan are well adapted to pediatric patients because of the small contact surface of the detectors and their high frequency and focus.
Real time definitely solves the technical problems caused by children's motion but the "single sweep" technique with B mode grey scale gives also very satisfactory images in children too small to cooperate.
No sedation is needed even in small patients or patients in poor physical condition but it is imperative for the echographist to be as calm as possible and for the surrounding room to be a quiet one.
If some patients are still too agitated to allow a good echogram, it is possible to plan the ultrasonic examination to coincide with the end of a sedation given for another purpose.
No preparation is needed but abdominal examination requires a few hours fasting and pelvic examination requires a full bladder.
The technical progress in ultrasound allows accurate measurement of the tumor size (diameters, contours and integration of the tumor surface in each space plane)

which enables to follow the rate of tumor growth or regression.
Two difficulties exists : air in the abdomen stops the
ultrasonic beam and renders the technique useless as far
as that specific area is concerned.
This occurs often in children : ileus caused by pain or
antineoplastic agents, or more simply large amount of
air swallowed because of fear.
Acoustic windows are thus used (liver, spleen, bladder)
to see as much of the abdominal cavity as possible in
supine position, kidneys being mainly examined in prone
position.
The other difficulty, when a tumor exists, is to compare
the same scanning planes on surveillance abdominal sonograms : the simplest solution consists of using abdominal topography (and reference as the xiphoid process,
ombilic, pubic bone) and consider the greatest tumor
diameter in a specific abdominal zone.

MATERIAL
        63 children with neoplastic disease were examined
echographically over a period of 2 years.  37 of these
children were on follow-up examination for a neoplasm
diagnosed previously.  The remaining 26 became sick during that 2 year period and had echograms shortly after
the onset of their clinical signs : ultrasounds confirmed the existence of a mass (or masses) and oriented the
further radiologic work up.
        The echography was repeated every 3 months to eva-
luate the size of their tumor, to look for metastases
and to track treatment complications.
        The different diagnosis of this serie figured as
follow :           I8 leukemia
                   I7 Wilms tumor
                   IO non Hodgkin lymphoma
                    5 neuroblastoma
                    3 Hodgkin disease
                    3 hepatoblastoma
                    2 rhabdomyosarcoma
                    I liposarcoma
                    I hemangioendothelioma
The correlation between clinical evaluation of the size
of the mass and ultrasound measurements was always satisfactory.
Ultrasound showed in two cases - one neuroblastoma and
one rhabdomyosarcoma - metastasis to the liver that were
not clinically suspected although the children were
known to have other secondary locations.

## DETECTION OF A NEOPLASTIC LESION AND EVALUATION OF ITS EXTENSION.

When an abdominal mass is suspected or palpated, ultrasonic examination of the abdomen and retroperitoneum should be the first imaging technique used to approach diagnosis.

Scouting the abdomen with the child in the supine position from the xiphoid process to the symphisis pubis and from flank to flank and then the retroperitoneal space in prone position will most of the time give the origin of the mass and its extension, and will help to decide which examinations to plan next in order to get complete information on the tumor.

Each abdominal organ should be examined as far as volume, echopattern, internal architecture and anatomical relationship with other organs and vessels are concerned and small amounts of ascitic fluid should be searched for.

### Case I

Hyperechogenic mass of the right flank in a five month old baby girl without margin between mass and liver tissue on the abdominal scan but with definite margin between mass and squeezed right kidney on both supine and prone scans.
The diagnosis of hepatoblastoma was confirmed by arteriography.

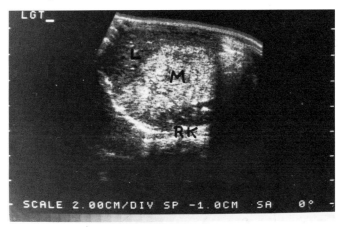

Fig.I.A. Sagittal scan on supine position hyperechogenic mass (M) within liver parenchyma (L). Flatened right kidney (RK)

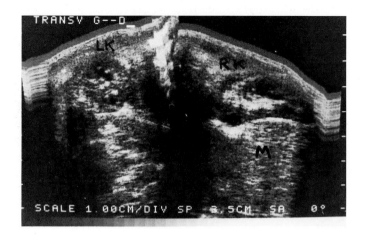

Fig.I.B. Transverse scan on prone position
Hyperechogenic mass (M) adjacent anteriorly and well limited from the right kidney (RK) Normal left kidney (LK).

Follow-up ultrasonic examination one year later
shows no signe of relapse.

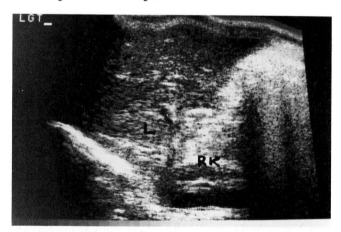

Fig.I.C. Sagittal scan in supine position
Right kidney (RK) behind right liver
lobe (L) of normal echopattern.

Case 2

Abdominal mass of approximately the same volume
and same hyperechogenic pattern as in Case I in
a I year old boy.
No anatomical limit between the mass and the
upper pole of the right kidney (the echofree
area within the mass may represent area of
necrosis or distorded calyces).

270

The IVP confirmed the presence of a Wilms tumor.

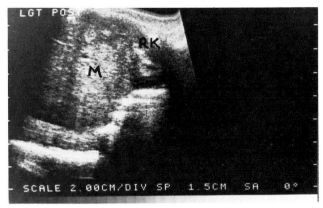

Fig.2.A. Sagittal scan in prone position
Hyperechogenic mass (M) emerging from
upper pole of right kidney (RK).

## Case 3

Diffuse abdominal pain and palpation of a mass
(or stools?) in the epigastric zone of a 2 year
old girl.
The sagittal and transverse scans show numerous
rather echofree masses scattered through the
abdomen,there is one mass bigger than the other
behind the bladder and another one with heterogeneous echopattern (high density echoes in the
center part encircled by a large zone of low
density echoes) at the level of the transverse
colon.

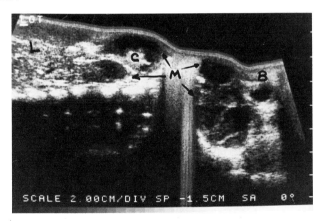

Fig.3.A. Sagittal scan in supine position
Numerous masses (M) with low echo pattern
between liver (L) and bladder (B). Transverse colon (C).

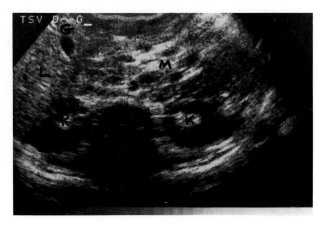

Fig.3.B. Transverse scan in supine position. Masses (M), liver (L), gallbladder
(G), kidneys (K).

A barium enema confirmed the existence of a non
hodgkin lymphoma and temporarily cured its
most common complication : the intussusception of
the last ileal loops (in this case at the level
of the transverse colon) accounting for the
"target" like ultrasonic image.

SEARCH FOR DISTANT METASTASIS OR OTHER TUMOR
LOCALISATION.

The role of correct staging of certain tumors or prompt
recognition of metastases is of increasing importance
for the planning of treatment, mostly to tailor its
agressiveness to the exact extension of the affected areas.

Lymphnodes : splanchnic and retroperitoneal lymphnode
chains are frequently involved in Hodgkin disease.
Lymphnodes can be visualized when enlarged either as
masses or indirectly by giving vascular compression.
Ultrasounds may therefore be of help in detecting lymphnodes enlargement in areas not reached by lymphography
and often poorly demonstrated by other techniques (for
ex. CAT scan)i.e. hepatic hilus, mesenteric artery ter-
ritory and pancreatic area in cases of Hodgkin or
lymphoma but also in case of any tumor producing lymphnode metastatic dissemination.

Case 3

Burkitt lymphoma in a 2 year old girl with
metastases closed to pancreatic tail.

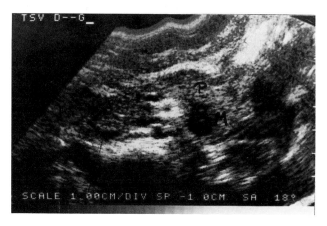

Fig.3.C. Transverse scan in supine position. Mass (M) at the level of pancreatic tail (P).

The liver
The parenchyma must be carefully examined when metastatic lesions are expected. Small echofree areas cr larger areas with borderline "mass compression" of the hepatic surrounding tissue should be looked for.

Case 4

Small echofree area within the liver that appeared during the course of treatment of a right suprarenal neuroblastoma in a 5 year old boy.

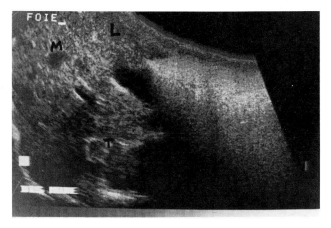

Fig.4.A. Sagittal scan in supine position Metastasis (M) within liver parenchyma (L) right suprarenal neuroblastoma (T).

Larger more echogenic metastasis with mass "compression" within the liver parenchyma.

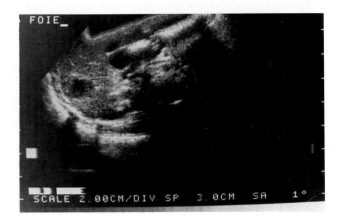

Fig.4.B. Transverse scan in supine position. Right liver lobe metastasis (M) of right suprarenal neuroblastoma.

## Inferior vena cava

The inferior vena cava must be examined thoroughly as much for extraluminal compressions as for metastatic material within its lumen.

## Kidneys

The presence of Wilms' tumor in the contralateral kidney should be looked for.

## RESPONSE TO TREATMENT AND FOLLOW-UP.

## Tumor volume

Measure devices either direct caliper or centimetric scales, or more recently echo computer for contours and surface integration, are of considerable interest in following growth or regression of a tumor and thus in encouraging to pursue or change therapy by relating tumor size to previous examination in the same patient.

### Case 5

Retroperitoneal liposarcoma in a 6 year old girl : heterogenous hyperechogenic mass measuring I05x54xII5mm. at the time of diagnosis.

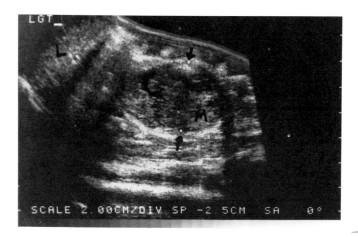

Fig.5.A. Sagittal scan in supine position. Liposarcoma of the retroperitoneum (M) with caliper measuring thickness (➡). Liver (L).

Dramatic growth of the mass during the 8 months
of survival : a few days before death, it measured I78x65xI37mm.

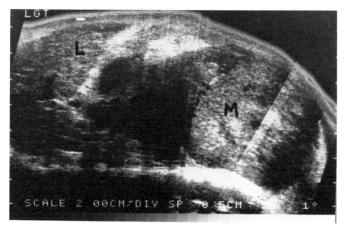

Fig.5.B. Same sagittal scanning plane
as in Fig.5.A. and same scale. Mass(M)
Liver (L).

## Case 6

Slow but continuous involution of an abdominal
Burkitt lymphoma originating from the mesenteric
root and including the mesenteric artery in a 6
year old girl.

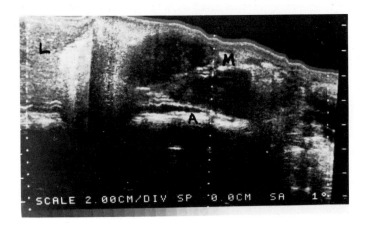

Fig.6.A. Sagittal scan in supine position.
Mass (M) measuring IO8x6Ox9Omm laminating
aorta (A). Liver (L).

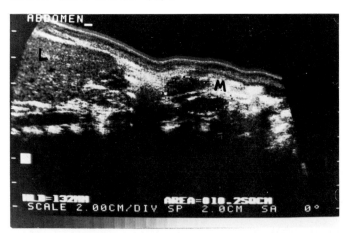

Fig.6.B. Same scanning plane, same scale,
one year later. Mass (M) measures 5Ix26
x43mm. Mass volume is IO.2 square cm.

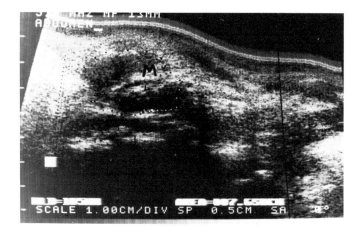

Fig.6.C. Same scanning plane, scale twice bigger than in Fig.6.B., 3 months later. Mass (M) measures 46x24x37mm. Mass volume has become 7.6 square cm.

## Case 7

Burkitt lymphoma of the right iliac fossa and pelvis in a II year old boy.

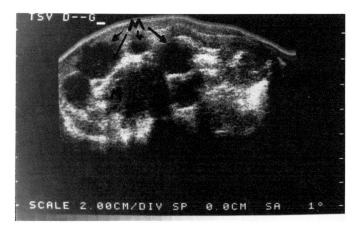

Fig.7.A. Transverse section in supine position of right iliac fossa showing multiple echofree masses (M).

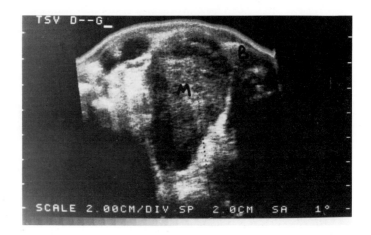

Fig.7.B. Transverse section of the pelvis : big lymphomatous mass (M) on the
right side of the bladder (B).
The mass measures 85xII7x70mm.

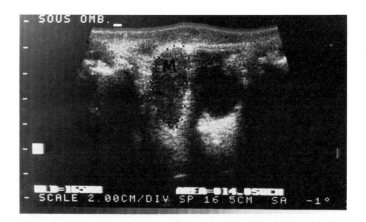

Fig.7.C. Transverse section of the pelvis, same scanning plane and same scale
as in Fig.7.B.  9 months later : the
mass (M) measures 6Ix66x3Imm.  The mass
volume has become I4.0 square cm.

Complications of treatment
They may be numerous but biliary and pancreatic complications are of particular interest for echographic
study because of easy recognition of pancreas and biliary tree.

278

## Case 8

Jaundice appearing during treatment of a Burkitt lymphoma in a 6 year old boy. Pancreatico duo-denal involvement and distal obstruction of the common bile duct by fibrosis following necrosis and regression of the tumor after radiotherapy.

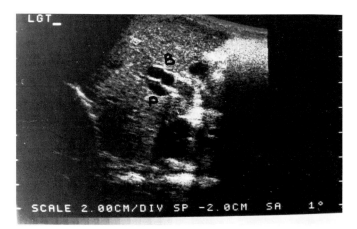

Fig.8.A. Sagittal scanning plane in supine position. Dilated common bile duct (B) above portal vein (P).

## Case 9

Detection of acute pancreatitis in a 3 year old child with ALL and treated with Asparaginase.

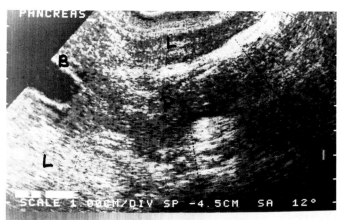

Fig.9.A. Transverse scan in supine posi-tion. Hyporeflective pancreas (P) that appears swollen - Liver (L) - Gallblad-der (B).

## CONCLUSION

Ultrasound appears to be an appropriate technique to follow the course of abdominal neoplastic disease in children.
In our experience there has always been a good correlation between technically satisfactory echograms and clinical findings. CAT and angiograms have been used preoperatively and for diagnostic purpose in a few instances.

## ACKNOWLEDGMENTS

We thank Mrs. N. Vanden Bossche and Mr. Y. Lammens for their friendly assistance in preparing the manuscript.

## REFERENCES.

I. Bernardino, M.E., and Green, B. : Ultrasonographic evaluation of chemotherapeutic response in hepatic metastases. Radiology I33, 437, I979.

2. Bree, R.L. and Green, B. : The gray scale sonographic appearence of intraabdominal mesenchymal sarcomas. Radiology I28, I93, I978.

3. Ferrucci, J.T.Jr.: Body ultrasonography. N. Engl.J. Med. 300, 538, I979.

4. Filly, R.A., Marglin, S. and Castellino, R.A. : The spectrum of subdiaphragmatic Hodgkin's disease and non Hodgkin's lymphoma. Cancer 38, 2I43, I976.

5. Filly, R. : Echography. In Parker B.R. and Castellino R.A., editors : Pediatric Oncologic Radiology, Saint Louis I977, the C.V. Mosby Co I03-I29.

6. Fleischer, A.C., Muhletaler, C.A. and James, A.E. : Sonographic patterns arising from normal and abnormal bowel. Radiologic Clin. of North America I8, I45, I980.

7. Green, B., Bree, R.L., Goldstein, H.M. and Stanley,C Gray scale ultrasound evaluation of hepatic neoplasms pattern and correlations. Radiology I24, 203, I977.

8. Kaplan, H.S. : Essentials of staging and management of the malignant lymphomas. Seminars in Roentgenology I5, 2I9, I980.

9. Kushner, D.C., Weinstein, H.J. and Kirkpatrick, J.A.: The radiologic diagnosis of leukemia and lymphoma in children. Seminars in Roentgenology I5, 3I6, I980.

280

10. Paling, M.R., Shawker, T.H. and Dwyer, A. : Ultra-
    sonic evaluation of therapeutic response in Tumors :
    its value and implications.  JCU 9, 281, 1981.

11. Shawker, T.H., Dunnick, N.R., Head, G.L. and
    Magrath, I.T. : Ultrasound evaluation of american
    Burkitt's lymphoma.  JCU 7, 279, 1979.

12. Tolbert, D.D., Zagzebski, J.A., Banjavic, R.A. and
    Wiley, A.L. : Quantitation of tumor volumes and
    response to therapy with ultrasound B.scans.
    Radiology 113, 705, 1974.

13. Wiener, S.N. and Parulekar, S.G. : Scintigraphy and
    ultrasonography of hepatic hemangioma.  Radiology 132,
    149, 1979.

# THE ULTRASONIC CHARACTERIZATION OF BREAST MALIGNANCIES

J. Jellins, T.S. Reeve[1], G. Kossoff and K. Griffiths

*Ultrasonics Institute, Sydney, NSW, Australia, [1]Department of Surgery, Royal North Shore Hospital, St. Leonards, NSW, Australia*

## INTRODUCTION

The development of high resolution grey scale ultrasonic scanners has provided the means to display morphological detail of the constituent tissues of the breast. The technique allows the visualization of both the texture and the distribution of the tissues in the breast and provides a basis for the recognition of abnormal tissue changes. The detection and diagnosis of malignant conditions relies on the identification of a number of characteristic features associated with particular disease processes and differentiating these features from the background detail present in the surrounding breast anatomy.

The breast is a difficult organ to interpret echographically due to the many variations in the normal patterns. In particular the interaction between the active breast tissue and the fatty tissue must be understood before serious attempts can be made in the detection and diagnosis of malignant conditions. Fatty tissue in the breast is always displayed with low level echoes which are similar in amplitude to those found in both benign and malignant lesions. The active breast tissue and supporting stroma are displayed with medium to high level echoes and are readily differentiated from regions of neoplastic changes.

## ECHOGRAPHIC FEATURES

A number of echographic features are present in malignant lesions and form part of the diagnostic criteria currently used in the detection and diagnosis of lesions. The implementation of the criteria in the interpretation of echograms provides a basis for recognizing pathological processes and in some instances classifying the lesions into histological groups. Simple and compound modes of scanning are required to reliably demonstrate all the features and the criteria are based on the availability of both types of echograms.

The criteria used in the classification of malignant lesions are listed in order of importance.

1. Distortion of breast architecture.
2. Internal echo content.
3. Skin involvement.
4. Boundary echoes.
5. Posterior detail.
6. Shape and position of mass.
7. Surrounding tissues.

The presence of malignant changes alters the physical structure of the breast parenchyma and causes a distortion of the breast architecture. In breast images this results in a low level echo region of discontinuity which is more readily recognized when surrounded by tissues producing medium to high level echoes. The discontinuity should extend over a number of levels and be commensurate with the size of the lesion.

The internal echo content of malignant lesions is variable but generally is displayed with echoes of low amplitude. The magnitude of the echoes in most instances is similar or less than those originating from fatty tissue and much less than the levels encountered from the breast parenchyma.

Changes in skin contour are readily visualized in echograms obtained with water path scanners. When associated with a well defined lesion, this feature reinforces its suspicious nature.

The presence of a skin change without the visualization of a lesion should be treated with extreme caution. This may be due to a malignancy which is either too small to be recognized or has insufficient ultrasonic features to be detected. A change in skin contour often results from previous incision and this should always be excluded.

The boundary echoes are not only related to the nature of the lesion but also to their inclination to the ultrasonic beam. The medial and lateral borders are visualized more readily than the anterior and posterior surfaces in most malignant lesions. Infiltrating lesions have characteristic jagged edge appearance but the presence of smooth boundaries should not exclude the possibility of a malignancy. This particularly applies to the less common forms of malignancies which may even be encapsulated. In some instances the boundary echoes are not demonstrated at all and the extent of the lesion can only be gauged by the contrast of the echoes from within the lesion with the echoes from the surrounding breast parenchyma. When boundary echoes are not well displayed in compound scanned echograms, simple scans from a number of different directions should be taken.

The display of the tissues posterior to the lesion is dependent on the composition of the contents of the lesion and is an important feature in differentiating between malignant and benign lesions. The posterior tissue may be displayed with an intensity similar to that of surrounding tissues or may be either reduced or intensified. The presence of a shadow behind a lesion with some doubtful features confirms its malignant nature as 2/3 of infiltrating carcinomas have this property. The remaining infiltrating duct carcinomas do not modify the posterior detail. Other less common carcinomas have either no effect on the posterior detail or may produce some degree of enhancement. Most carcinomas greater than 2cm do not alter the posterior detail.

The shape and position of the lesion are related to its pathology. Most malignancies are irregular in shape and located within the breast parenchyma. With increase in size of the lesions the shape is partially determined by the surrounding tissues and may become more irregular. Advanced lesions occupy space outside of the parenchyma and often invade the subcutaneous tissues or pectoralis muscles.

The surrounding tissues react to the presence of malignancies by becoming fibrotic and are then displayed with higher level echoes. Malignancies which are enclosed by a capsule tend to compress the surrounding tissues giving them an appearance which is more dense than usual.

Characteristics found in the more common malignancies are shown in the table below.

|  | INFILTRATING DUCT | ADENOCARCINOMA | MEDULLARY |
|---|---|---|---|
| FEATURES | Characteristic | Less Characteristic | More Distinct |
| INTERNAL ECHO CONTENT | Very Low to Low | Low to medium | Very Low |
| SKIN INVOLVEMENT | Frequent Involvement | Unaffected | Protrusion |
| BOUNDARY ECHOES | Jagged | Less Jagged | Well Demarcated |
| POSTERIOR DETAIL | Shadowed | Unaffected | Enhanced |
| SHAPE | Irregular | Irregular | Irregular |
| SURROUNDING TISSUES | Reactive | Unaffected | Unaffected |
| APPEARANCE | Indrawn | Localised | Expansive |

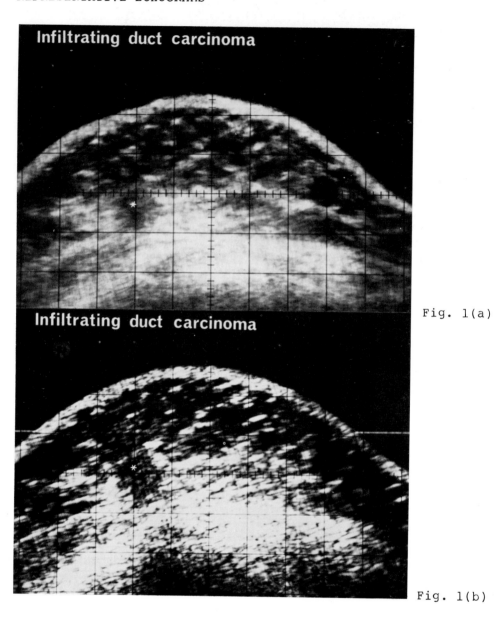

Fig. 1(a)

Fig. 1(b)

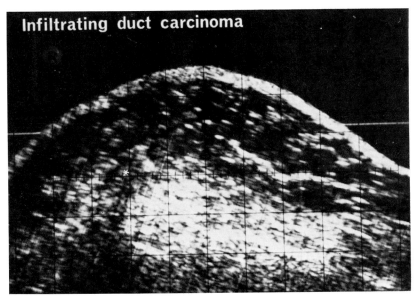

Infiltrating duct carcinoma

Fig. 1(c)

Figure 1(a).  A compound scanned echogram with a well defined 1.5cm infiltrating duct carcinoma.  The internal echo content is displayed with low level echoes similarly to the amplitude of echoes in the subcutaneous fatty tissue.  There is evidence of skin retraction immediately superiorly to the tumour.  The boundaries are jagged.  The high level echoes surrounding the tumour are consistent with the presence of reactive fibrotic tissue.  Many infiltrating duct carcinomas have an indrawn appearance.  The central portion of the tumour in this echogram and all subsequent echograms with malignancies has been marked with an asterisk.

Figure 1(b).  A simple scan of the same section with the transducer tilted does not show shadowing of posterior detail.

Figure 1(c).  A simple scan of the same section with the transducer tilted in a different direction shows shadowing of posterior detail.

|              | MUCOID       | LOBULAR            | ANAPLASTIC     |
|--------------|--------------|--------------------|----------------|
| FEATURES     | Distinct     | Less Distinct      | Less Distinct  |
| INTERNAL ECHO CONTENT | Variable | Very Low to low | Variable |
| SKIN INVOLVEMENT | Thickening | Unaffected      | Unaffected     |
| BOUNDARY ECHOES | Less Jagged | Not Evident      | Indistinct     |
| POSTERIOR DETAIL | Unaffected | Unaffected      | Unaffected     |
| SHAPE        | Irregular    | Irregular          | Irregular      |
| SURROUNDING TISSUES | Unaffected | Unaffected    | Unaffected     |
| APPEARANCE   | Localised    | Invasive           | Inconclusive   |

The differentiation of malignancies from benign
conditions is essential in the assessment of patients
with breast disease. Benign conditions may have some of
the ultrasonic features found in malignancies and these
should be recognized in order to avoid a high number of
false positive interpretations in those areas where a
malignancy is suspected.

Conditions which mimic the appearance of neoplastic
lesions are often seen in patients undergoing
involutional changes. The areas of fatty deposition are
difficult to differentiate from more sinister conditions
and generally occur in those patients in age groups
where the risk of a malignancy is lower. Fibroadenomas
are often displayed in the ultrasonic images similarly
to the areas of fatty deposition but with better defined
boundaries.

The characteristics associated with these benign
changes are shown in the table.

|                        | FATTY INFILTRATION | FIBROADENOMAS                     |
|------------------------|--------------------|-----------------------------------|
| INTERNAL ECHO CONTENT  | Low                | Variable                          |
| SKIN INVOLVEMENT       | Uninvolved         | Uninvolved                        |
| BOUNDARY ECHOES        | Not Present        | Smooth Prominent Anterior Border  |
| POSTERIOR DETAIL       | Enhanced           | Variable                          |
| SHAPE                  | Irregular          | Regular                           |
| SURROUNDING TISSUES    | Unaffected         | Unaffected                        |

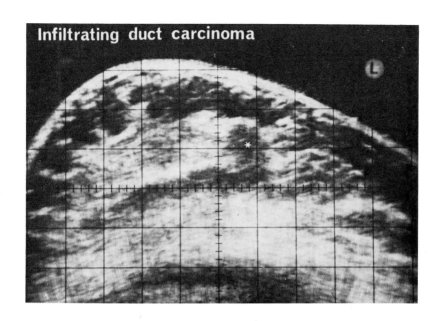

Figure 2. A 1.5 x 2cm region of disrupted architecture within the breast parenchyma is shown in this image. The amplitude of echoes from this region is lower than that of the surrounding tissue and higher than that from the subcutaneous fatty tissue. The boundary echoes are jagged and the shape of the lesion is irregular.

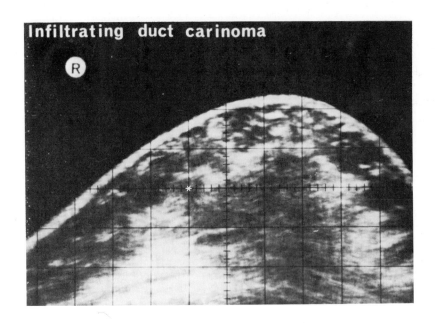

Figure 3. The echogram of the right breast contains a
1cm infiltrating duct carcinoma situated superficially
in the breast parenchyma. The tumour contains low level
echoes and its boundaries are jagged. There is no
evidence of skin involvement or shadowing of posterior
detail with this tumour. Situated medially to the
tumour is a 5 x 4cm region of somewhat similar
appearance due to involutional changes.

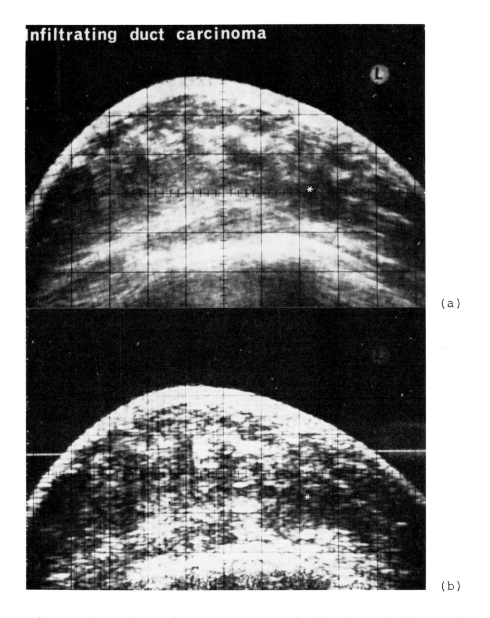

Infiltrating duct carcinoma

(a)

(b)

Figure 4. These images show an indistinct infiltrating duct carcinoma obtained with both (a) compound and (b) simple scanned echograms. The tumour is approximately 2cm in diameter and has boundaries which are less distinct than those visualised in the previous examples. The medial margin of the tumour is better demonstrated on a simple scan.

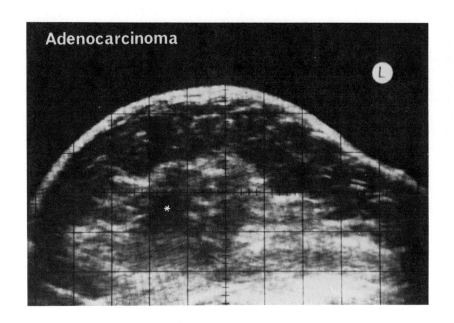

Figure 5. Adenocarcinoma measuring 4 x 3cm containing low to medium level echoes of higher amplitude than those in the subcutaneous fat. The boundaries although not well displayed are jagged. With this type of tumour there is no change in the display of the posterior detail.

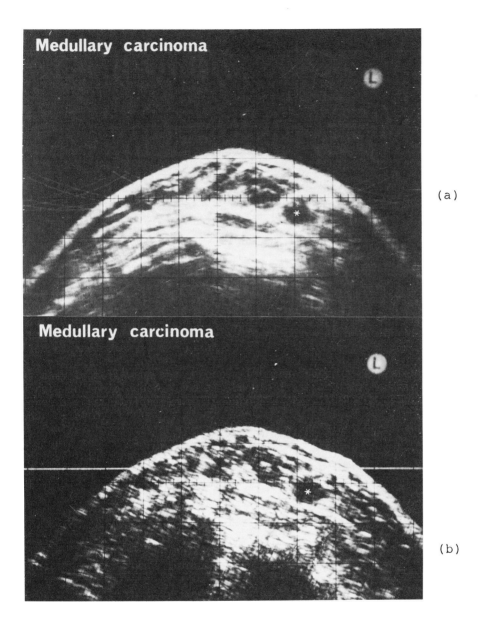

Figure 6. Medullary carcinomas are more distinctive than either infiltrating duct carcinomas or adenocarcinomas. Both the compound (a) and simple (b) scans show the central region with very low to low level echoes. This type of carcinoma is well demarcated from the surrounding tissues. The posterior detail is enhanced being displayed with high level echoes. The appearance of medullary carcinomas suggests that the tumour is expansive in nature rather than invasive.

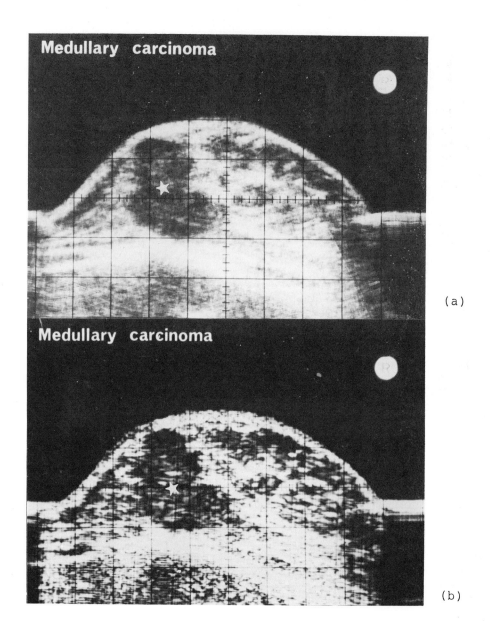

(a)

(b)

Figure 7. An advanced medullary carcinoma measuring 2.5 x 3.8cm with an irregular shape is shown in these images (a) and (b). The echoes from within the tumour are predominantly low in amplitude but there is evidence of isolated medium to high level echoes. The tumour has caused some skin protrusion.

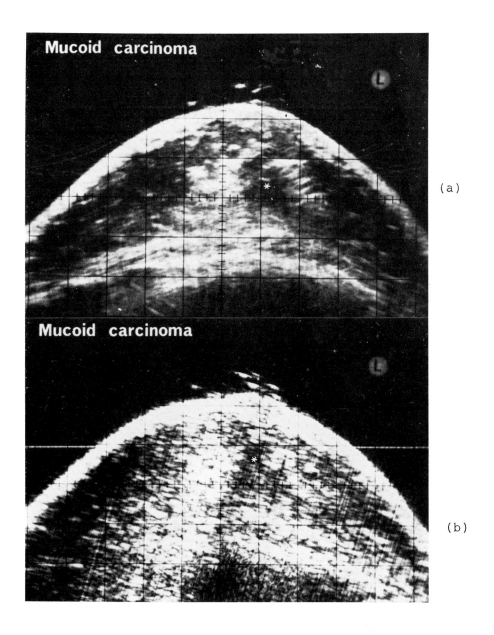

Mucoid carcinoma

(a)

Mucoid carcinoma

(b)

Figure 8. Mucoid carcinomas are less easily recognisable due to their variable internal echo content. The level of the echoes from within the tumour is similar to the echoes from the subcutaneous fatty tissues. Skin thickening can be often demonstrated but these changes are subtle and may be better visualised on simple scans. The compound echogram (a) shows the tumour more clearly than the simple scan (b).

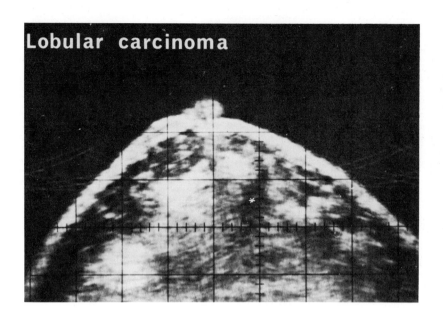

Figure 9. Lobular carcinomas are less distinct in their appearance. The tumour can be recognised by the contrast of the low level internal echoes to the higher level echoes from the surrounding tissues. With this type of tumour the boundary echoes are not always demonstrated. The shape is irregular and is consistent with an invasive process.

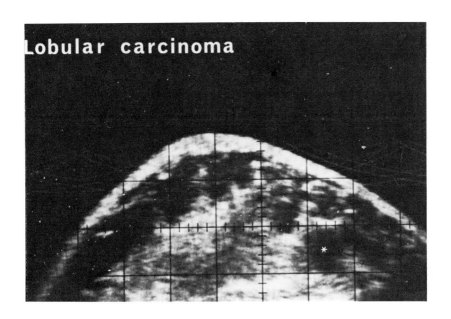

Figure 10. The lobular carcinoma contains very low level internal echoes giving an appearance similar to that obtained with some liquid filled lesion. The boundaries of this 1.5cm tumour are irregular and not well displayed. The surrounding breast architecture is distorted consistent with the presence of malignancy.

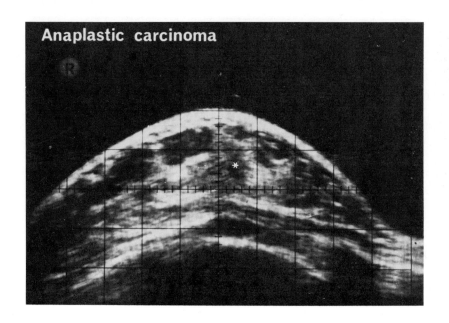

Figure 11. The echogram shows an anaplastic carcinoma situated in the middle portion of the breast. The internal echo content is variable. The boundaries are jagged and uneven. The disruption of the breast architecture is gross.

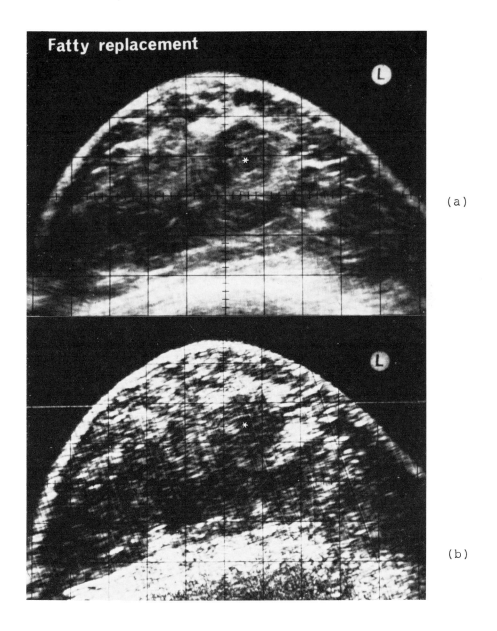

**Fatty replacement**

(a)

(b)

Figure 12. Areas of fatty replacement are displayed as low level echo regions within the breast parenchyma. In some cases the high level echoes from the glandular and the fibrotic tissues appear to encapsulate these regions (marked with an asterisk) giving the echographic appearance of a tumour. This is well demonstrated in the compound scan (a) and the simple scan (b).

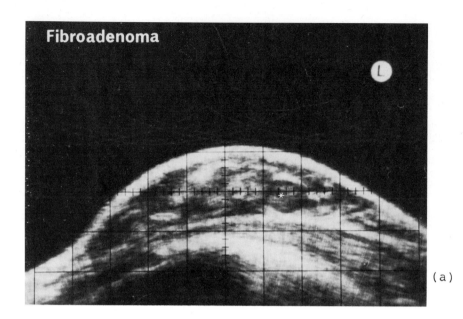

Fibroadenoma

(a)

Figure 13. Benign lesions with low echo content and
well demarcated boundaries can appear similar to
malignancies. The internal echo content of this
fibroadenoma is homogeneous with medium level echoes
which are more even in distribution than seen with
cancers. Fibroadenomas have smooth boundaries which are
not visualized with malignant lesions. The boundaries
are better demonstrated in the compound scan (a) than in
the simple scan (b)

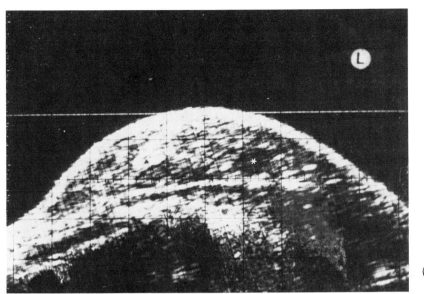

(b)

## RESULTS

The application of the diagnostic criteria for the detection and diagnosis of malignancies shows that for tumours greater than 5mm in diameter, the sensitivity of the technique is 83%. This has been established in the examination of over 4000 patients of which 147 at biopsy were proven to be cancers. The most common form of malignancy in this series was found to be in the infiltrating duct carcinoma of which there were 114. These tumours are well demarcated from the surrounding tissues and the boundaries mostly jagged, approximately 67% shadow the posterior detail. Twelve adenocarcinomas were visualized and the echographic appearance of these tumours has been variable. The internal echo content is lower than that found with the adipose tissue and the boundaries are more regular in appearance than those found with the infiltrating duct carcinomas. Six medullary carcinomas have been visualized and although these tumours are well demarcated from the surrounding tissues, their attenuation characteristics are less and thus these carcinomas have less distinct features and these include such types of mucoid (6), lobular (4) and anaplastic (5).

## CONCLUSION

Ultrasound can be used as an imaging modality in the detection and diagnosis of malignancies greater than 1cm in diameter. With these tumours the echographic characteristics are sufficiently distinct to enable differing ultrasonic patterns to be assigned to the various forms of malignancies. This allows the clinician not only the opportunity to detect and diagnose the tumour but in some cases from its ultrasonic appearance recognise the type of malignancy.

## REFERENCES

1. Jellins, J., Kossoff, G., Reeve, T.S. and Barraclough, B.H. (1975) Ultrasonic grey scale visualisation of breast disease. Ultrasound Med. Biol. 1: 393-404.
2. Jellins, J., Kossoff, G. and Reeve, T.S. (1975) Current and potential capabilities of ultrasound imaging for breast cancer diagnosis. Proc. Society of Photo-Optical Instrumentation Engineers, 70. Medicine IV 372-374.

3.  Kossoff, G., Jellins, J. and Reeve, T.S. (1976)
    Ultrasound in the detection of early breast cancer.
    Recent results in Cancer Research, VIII
    International Symposium, Dusseldorf, June 1976.
4.  Reeve, T.S., Jellins, J., Kossoff, G. and
    Barraclough, B.H. (1978) Ultrasonic visualisation
    of breast cancer. Aust. N.Z. J. Surg., Vol. 48,
    No. 3, 278.
5.  Jellins, J., Reeve, T.S., Croll, J. and Kossoff, G.
    (1982) Results of Breast Echographic Examinations
    in Sydney, Australia 1972-1979. Seminars in
    Ultrasound, March 1982 (In press).

# EXPERIENCE WITH SONOGRAPHIC DIAGNOSIS OF BREAST CANCER IN A DIAGNOSTIC BREAST CLINIC

Joan Croll

*Clinical Director, Sydney Square Diagnostic Breast Clinic, Sydney Square, Sydney, NSW, Australia*

Breast cancer is the commonest cancer in Australian women, and the leading cause of death between the ages of 40 and 54. There has been no apparent decrease in mortality from this disease, despite great advances in the treatment of cancer in other sites. Patients with breast symptoms must be adequately investigated so that those who have breast cancer may be diagnosed before hospital admission. Equally importantly, those who do not have breast cancer may be correctly reassured without the need for open biopsy. The cost-effectiveness of adequate investigation of breast symptoms is both financial and emotional. In order to arrive at a correct diagnosis in any one patient the tests should be tailored to suit the need.

The Sydney Square Diagnostic Breast Clinic was established as a 'model' to test the individual contributions of surgical opinion, film-screen mammography, xeromammography, water-bath echography of the whole breast and fine-needle aspiration cytology, in the investigation of patients referred with breast problems.

MATERIALS AND METHODS.

During a three year- period, (April 1978 – June 1981), 7500 women with breast symptoms have been referred to the Clinic for investigation and an opinion. The family physician or family planning clinic referred 85% and the remainder were referred by specialist surgeons and gynaecologists.

The first 1500 patients formed a pilot study to test methods and data collection formats. The age of patients has ranged from a 10 year-old girl with unilateral breast development to a 91 year-old woman with nipple discharge. The average age of patients is 43 years. The Clinic is a non-profit organisation established by a Sydney philanthropist, and each patient pays on a fee-for-service basis, according to their health insurance cover.

The patient remains the responsibility of her referring doctor, who is informed of Clinic opinion by

The financial support of the A W Tyree Foundation is gratefully acknowledged.

305

Table 1. Symptomatology of a sample of 500 consecutive patients referred for investigation of a breast problem

| SYMPTOMATOLOGY | % of clinic popn |
|---|---|
| lump | 38.0% # |
| pain | 24.0% |
| lumpy | 8.0% |
| nple disch, invsn | |
| itchy, ulcerated | 8.0% |
| thickening | 7.0% |
| enlgement | 4.0% |
| mam abnormality | 3.0% |
| risk factors | 3.0% |
| cancerphobia | 2.0% |
| none | 2.0% |
| prev mastectomy | 0.5% |
| skin change | 0.5% |
| | 100.0% |

# 4% of these patients had cancer

telephone when urgent treatment is recommended, and by full written report in any case.

All patients are examined by one of 45 consultant surgeons who attend Clinic sessions on a rostered basis. Two surgeons are present each day, and second surgical opinion is sought in all cases with a suspicious clinical, mammographic or ultrasonic lesion.

Mammography has been performed on women over 25 years using a CGR Senomax for both film-screen and/or xeromammography. More recently a CGR Senograph 500T equipped with a 1 in 5 moving grid system has been used for film-screen mammography only. Xeromammography proved to be less reliable than the film technique in our hands. Routine cranio-caudad and medio-lateral oblique views are taken. In addition ,latero-medial views are taken to demonstrate a medial lesion, and 90° laterals to localise an impalpable lesion or microcalcifications, when necessary. Mammograms are read by the radiologist present on the day, and again by the author. In equivocal cases, three or more opinions are sought on the films.

Ultrasonography is performed on all women under 25 years and they are not examined by mammography except in exceptional circumstances. Ultrasonography is used in most older women and in all those who have a clinical or mammographic lesion or dense, dysplastic breasts. The test is performed with an UI Octoson dedicated to breast work equipped with 4 MHz transducers. Images are recorded on 9-format film using a Dunn camera, and a detailed explanation of our methods follows.

The sonographer examines the patient and takes a brief history, marking scars from previous biopsy or skin lesions on relevant diagrams. After explaining the test to the patient, neutral detergent solution is sponged onto the skin to reduce surface tension and the entire breast is immersed in the water-bath, which is kept at a constant temperature of 35°C. The left breast is examined first so that the patient may observe the screen which helps to allay anxiety. Relaxation is essential as movement may disturb the clarity and definition of the images.

The nipple is centred on Y-000, then the transducer arm is moved to the upper limit of breast tissue. Using compound scans, sections are taken at 5mm intervals down to the lower limit of breast tissue. Areas of interest are noted and sections down to 1mm are performed to identify the boundary and internal echo content of the lesion when first visualised. Simple scans are done later to check for enhancement or shadowing of posterior detail.

Rotation markers are placed through any areas of interest, and the gantry turned 90° to take sections at right angles. Simple scans from varying angles are conducted through any area of interest. The examination takes a minimum of 20 minutes, and longer if particular attention is paid to an area of interest.

In this Clinic, for reasons of time, routine sagittal cuts of the unaffected breast are not performed. We rely on the experience of the sonographer to be alerted to an area of possible suspicion while performing the routine transerve scans. It is accepted that this is not an 'ideal' situation, however experience has shown this method to be a practical application of the test in our circumstances.

Compression of the breast during examination has recently been introduced in those patients with palpable lesions which have not been well-demonstrated, and in those with sonographically 'difficult' breasts. Compression causes problems with orientation of any lesion seen, as it is not possible to centre the nipple as described above, and breast anatomy is distorted. Compression has however, added valuable information in some solid lesions, giving better definition of border characteristics, and internal echo content.

Ultrasonography is not performed on all patients presenting to the Clinic because of the time factor, as each test takes at least twenty minutes to complete. Should an area of clinical interest require sagittal sections and further simple scans as a source of greater information, the test may take considerably longer.

Newer developments presently being tested in Australia and elsewhere using different recording techniques, may cut the testing time considerably. However, we are accustomed to the quality of the images given by our machine, and particularly appreciate the ability to compare all sections of both breasts on the viewing box concurrently. Although video-recording appears to be an attractive alternative, the ability to compare a particular frame from one breast with the identical frame in the other may not be available. Such comparisons are essential when comparing skin outline for example.

Ultrasonography is performed routinely in those patients with clinical masses, non-specific mammographic masses, and in patients with dysplastic breasts.

FINE-NEEDLE ASPIRATION CYTOLOGY

Fine needle aspiration is performed on cysts which are more than 1 to 2 cms in diameter, whether detected clinically or sonographically. This not only confirms the diagnosis, but also treats the condition.

Fine-needle aspiration biopsy of solid lesions is performed as a diagnostic test using a 23 to 25 gauge needle and 10cc syringe. Several passes are made at different angles into the lesion with suction applied by a Franzen handle. Alcohol-fixed, air-dried and cyto-spin specimens are prepared for histological examination.

COMBINED OPINION

Although all tests are read 'blind' in the first instance, the consultants discuss their findings together before reporting the combined opinion to the patient and the referring doctor. It is essential to correlate mammography with echography for instance, as an apparent sonographic mass may prove to be an area of entrapped fat which is well demonstrated mammographically. Letters detailing the results of the examinations and the combined opinion of the consultant specialists are sent to the referring doctor in all cases.

TRAINING OF TECHNICIAN AND INTERPRETING PHYSICIAN.

Considerable training time is required for this test to be performed with confidence, and we have found that technicians with a sound knowledge of breast anatomy and/or mammography are able to learn breast echography more quickly than those without such knowledge. Likewise a reporting physician who is an experienced mammographer will learn to report more quickly, and his reading will be more accurate than the reading of a non-mammographer.

FOLLOW-UP OF PATIENTS

Information on patients with suspicious results is sought by telephone and letter. This Clinic is not attached to a hospital or university, and patients are referred for an opinion from widely scattered areas. Biopsies on our patients have been performed by more than 75 different surgeons, and histology has been reported by many different pathologists. Despite these difficulties, we have 100% follow-up in those patients in whom a suspicious lesions was reported on combined opinion. Follow-up to establish false negative opinion is even more difficult. We have recently compared our patient population with names of patients with breast cancer registered with the NSW Cancer Registry. For the purposes of this paper, only those patients with histologically proven breast cancer who were examined by grey-scale echography using the Octoson will be discussed. One hundred and ninety patients with proven breast cancer, 76% of our cancer population, fit into this category.

RESULTS.

SONOGRAPHY COMPARED WITH SURGICAL OPINION.

In patients with breasts described by the examining surgeon as 'normal' or 'diffuse benign disease', that is those in whom no tumour was felt, ultrasonography demonstrated a solid lesion or an area of suspicion in 11 of 14 cases. It is important to note that the impalpability of tumours is not necessarily because they are characterised by mammographic microcalcifications or are too small to feel, but also because the lesion may be deeply placed, or be within very active breast tissue, in which palpation is not easy.

Table 2. Results of breast echography in patients with proven breast cancer which was not palpated.

| NUMBER PATIENTS | SONOGRAPHY | | | |
|---|---|---|---|---|
| | positive | suspicious | negative | total |
| 14 | 7 | 4 | 3 | 14 |

In patients in whom a palpable lesion was thought to be clinically benign, but in whom cancer was later confirmed by histology, ultrasonography was reported as positive in 10 of the 20 instances.

Table 3. Results of breast echography in patients with proven breast cancer in whom surgical opinion was reported as a benign mass.

| NUMBER PATIENTS | SONOGRAPHY | | | |
|---|---|---|---|---|
| | positive | suspicious | negative | total |
| 20 | 10 | 0 | 9 | 19* |

* ultrasound was reported as unsatisfactory in one patient because the technician had not taken cuts sufficiently high above nipple to demonstrate the palpable cancer in the axillary tail of Spence.

As stated earlier it is only possible for the interpreting physician to report on those images supplied to him by his technician. As in mammography, examination of the patient by the technician performing the test is essential if palpable lesions are to be demonstrated.

In patients with palpable lesions recorded as 'probably benign' by the examing surgeons, in whom cancer was later proven histologically, ultrasonography was positive or suspicious in 13 of the 17 cases.

Table 4. Results of breast echography in patients with proven breast cancer in which surgical opinion reported a 'probably benign' mass.

| NUMBER PATIENTS | SONOGRAPHY | | | |
|---|---|---|---|---|
| | positive | suspicious | negative | total |
| 17 | 10 | 3 | 4 | 17 |

The remainder of the patients with proven breast cancer, 136 out of 190 or 72%, were reported as suspicious or frankly malignant lesions on clinical examination. Ultrasonography demonstrated postive or suspicious signs in 80% of these patients with clinical cancers.

FALSE NEGATIVE ULTRASONOGRAPHY

Ultrasonography is most accurate in mammographically dense breast tissue. It is therefore an ideal complement for mammography because mammography is least accurate in dense breast tissue. Conversely, ultrasonography frequently fails to demonstrate a mass lesion in a fatty breast despite an obvious clinical and mammographic cancer, because the echoes recorded from such tumours are similar in amplitude to those recorded from fatty tissue.

Table 5. False negative sonograms and mammograms compared with the mammographic classification of breast parenchyma in 180 patients with proven breast cancer.

| PARENCHYMA | 24 FALSE NEGATIVE MAMMOGRAMS | 32 FALSE NEGATIVE SONOGRAMS |
|---|---|---|
| atrophic | 8% | 56% * |
| mild dysplasia | 42% | 23% |
| marked dyspasia | 25% | 9% |
| moderate ductal | 17% | 3% |
| marked ductal | 8% | 9% |
| | 100% | 100% |

* This percentage would be higher if sonography had been performed on all patients with atrophic breasts who had obvious mammographic cancers.

310

We do not perform sonography in patients with atrophic breasts, unless a non-specific mammographic or clinical lesion requires elucidation.

The most common sonographic evidence of malignancy when using the water-bath technique is disturbance of the skin-line. With the breast dependent in the water-bath, areas of skin flattening or retraction are dramatically demonstrated. The strands of fibrous tissue associated with scirrous carcinomata, cause skin distortion in the dependent breast in many cases before these changes become clinically or mammographically detectable.

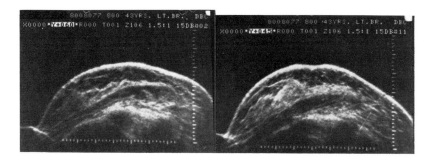

Figure 1. Demonstrates skin flattening in Y+060 and skin dimpling in Y+045, without obvious underlying mass . This patient had no discrete clinical or mammographic lesion, but carcinoma was proven by biopsy.

Skin flattening and/or thickening has been seen in patients with mammographic microcalcifications without associated mass, often when no palpable lesion is present.

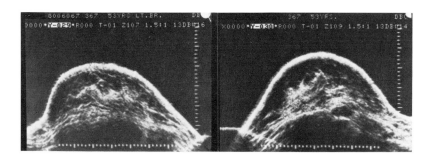

Figure 2. Note skin flattening in Y-029 in left breast, obvious when compared to Y-030 right breast. Patient aged 53 had clinical Paget's disease of nipple,but extensive intraduct carcinoma within the breast was not palpable.

Skin-line is distorted by the application of compression, so that all patients are examined with the breast dependent initially, and compression is applied should it be indicated, only after these images have been recorded.

Areas of low-level ehoes which are suspicious for carcinoma are usually well demonstrated in dense breast tissue, but compression of the breast will gives better definition of mass outlines and internal echo content.

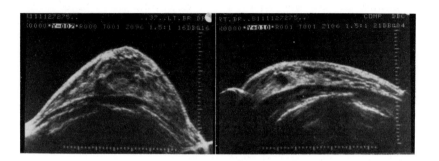

Figure 3. Demonstrates a suspicious area of low-level echoes in Y-007 in the dependent breast. Compression was applied with polythene wrap and the scan repeated. In Y+010 the irregular area of low-evel echoes is seen more clearly, and arouses greater suspicion. Note: The position of the lesion is disturbed by compression.

As Jellins has discussed the sonographic appearances of malignancy elsewhere in this issue (1), no definitve statements are made in this paper, but several technical procedures have been illustrated and discussed in detail.

DISCUSSION

In the experience of this Clinic, ultrasonography of the breast is not a stand-alone test. Correlation with recent mammography and clinical examination is essential in symptomatic patients aged 25 or older.

Ultrasonography and mammography are complementary tests and when one test is more likely to produce a false negative, the other is more likely to produce a true positive result, as illustrated in Table 5.

When a patient has been reassured, after adequate testing, that there is no evidence of carcinoma at the time of Clinic visit, this opinion has been proven correct 99.95% of cases. As discussed earlier in this paper, one cancer has been histologically confirmed in every 1.6 biopsies when the lesion was thought to be suspicious.

One cancer has been proven in each one hundred biopsies which were recommended for a lesion thought to be benign on combined opinion.

We have found that ultrasonography of the breast has prevented many benign biopsies which may have been performed for non-specific clinical or mammographic lesions. The ability of this test to differentiate between cystic and solid lesions has also been discussed elsewhere in this publication. The usefulness of such definitive information in a diagnostic clinic such as this, cannot be too greatly emphasised. The usefulness of ultrasonography in patients with cancer has been shown in tables 1 to 5. When compared to surgical opinion in these patients, sonography has proven to be more accurate.

ACKNOWLEDGEMENTS. Ultrasonography results reported in this paper have been interpreted by Dr Vic Wong Doo, Dr Richard Picker, Dr Bruce Barraclough, Dr James Ryan and by the author. Sonography has been performed by Jane Kotevich, Jan Waddington and Margaret Tabrett.

Thanks are due to my daughter Elisabeth for her work in collation and processing of the data from this Clinic.

REFERENCES:

1. Jellins, Jack: The ultrasonic characteristics of malignancies. Excerpta Medica — First International Symposium on Ultrasound and Cancer, Brussels, July 1982.

# SCREENING OF BREAST CANCER BY ECHOGRAPHY

T. Wagai and M. Tsutsumi

*Medical Ultrasonics Research Center, Juntendo University School of Medicine, Hongo, Bunkyo-ku, Tokyo, Japan*

Together with technological improvement of echographic equipments, echographic examination of the breast has been widely utilized for the detection of breast cancer with it's improved diagnostic accuracy. For instance, as the pulse echo method, not only simple and compound mechanical scanning technique with water-pass method but also B-mode and C-mode imaging techniques by applying linear array realtime scanner have been developed. At the same time, various new techniques such as the transmission imaging i.e. ultrasonic holography and ultrasonic computed tomography ( CT ) and the ultrasonic Doppler imaging have been applied practically for the imaging of breast tissue. Early detection of breast cancer is very important from the point of clinical treatment and screening of breast cancer had been actively carried out by using X-ray mammography, xerography, thermography, echography and others. Since the hazard problems of X-ray mammography was discussed for the screening of breast cancer, echography has been noticed and expected as a tool of screening with it's excellent diagnostic accuracy and various clinical advantages. In this paper, present status of detecting breast cancer by echography and of screening by echography which have been performed at the Research Center are reported.

EQUIPMENT FOR ECHOGRAPHIC BREAST IMAGING AND ECHOGRAPHIC IMAGES OF BREAST LESIONS

After the development of various scanning modalities for the echographic imaging of the breast such as simple linear, arc and compound scanning techniques, the water coupling mechanical linear scanner has been developed at the Research Center ( Fig.5 ) and routinely used with it's excellent echographic image quality, compact design and easy clinical procedure. Concaved PZT and recently PVDF transducer with 5 or 7.5MHz are applied. The scanning stroke is 15cm and scanning speed is two second and serial parallel echography with any desired interval are recorded. Depth of water in the water bag is 5 to 10cm.
Besides such equipment, new ultrasonic imaging techniques such as digital realtime imaging, ultrasonic holography and ultrasonic CT have been also investigated from

the point of clinical efficacy at the Research Center. Following, several examples of echographic images of breast lesions obtained by simple linear scanning modality.

Fig.1 is an example of fibrocystic disease obtained by simple linear and compound scanning technique at the same case. Although the compound scanning technique is theoretically ideal for obtaining more faithful echographic images than simple scanning technique, artifact phenomena accompanied with scanning modality have to be considered. Fig.2 is four cases of medullary tubular carcinoma. Irregular, lobulated and expanded margin with irregular internal echo content are characteristic and images of necrotic change are detected often in this type of carcinoma. Fig.3 is four cases of scirrhous carcinoma. Irregular, spiculated or sharply-edged margin with fine uniform internal echo content are characteristic in scirrhous carcinoma. Acoustic posterior shadowing is mainly detected in this type of carcinoma. Although papillo-tubular carcinoma showes malignant appearance with irregular margin and internal echo content, characteristic feature is not so clear compared with other type of carcinoma.

As the result of echographic differentiation of breast tumors which were experienced at the Research Center during the last 8 years is shown in the Table. Diagnostic accuracy on 232 cases of cancer was 88.3% and it was almost same with that of X-ray mammography. Scirrhous carcinoma showed better diagnostic accuracy ( 91.3% ) than other type of carcinoma and diagnostic accuracy of early carcinoma belongs to $T_1$ ( TNM classification ) was 80.7%. Differentiation

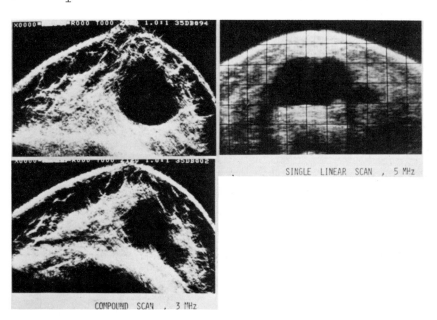

Fig.1   Echographic images of mammary cyst by compound scanning(3MHz) and simple linear scanning (5MHz)

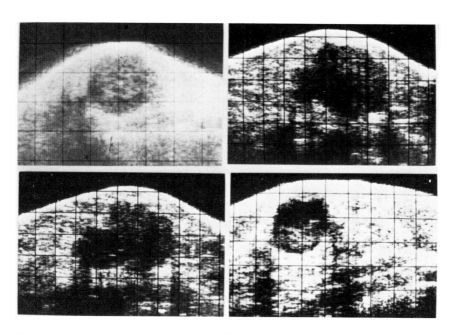

Fig.2 Echographic images of medullary tubular carcinoma by linear
      scanning ( 5MHz )

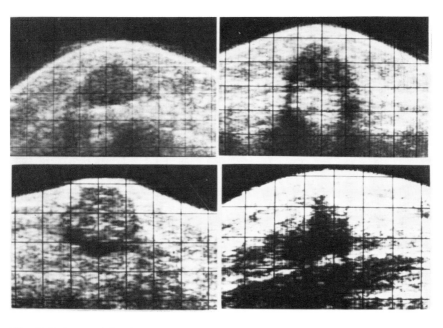

Fig.3 Echographic images of scirrhous carcinoma by linear scanning
                                                    ( 5MHz )

ECHOGRAPHIC DIAGNOSIS OF BREAST CARCINOMA
232 cases   Juntendo University Hospital 1973- '80

| Histology | | Echographic image | | % |
|---|---|---|---|---|
| scirrhous carcinoma | 81 | malig.appear. | 74 | 91.3 |
| med.tub.carcinoma | 96 | malig.appear. | 85 | 88.5 |
| pap.tub.carcinoma | 33 | malig.appear. | 27 | 81.8 |
| others | 22 | malig.appear. | 19 | 86.3 |
| Total | 232 | malig.appear. | 205 | 88.3 |
| $T_1$ | 52 | malig.appear | 42 | 80.7 |
| $T_2$ | 136 | malig.appear. | 122 | 89.7 |
| $T_{3-4}$ | 44 | malig.appear. | 41 | 93.1 |

DIAGNOSIS OF BREAST TUMORS BY ECHOGRAPHY AND MAMMOGRAPHY
Juntendo University, 1970- '80

| | mammography | | echography | |
|---|---|---|---|---|
| malig.tumors 232 | malig.appear. | 192(82.7%) | 205 | (88.3%) |
| | susp.malig.appear. | 34(14.6%) | 18 | ( 7.7%) |
| | no malig.appear | 6( 2.5%) | 9 | ( 3.8%) |
| benign tumors 612 | no malig.appear. | 540(88.2%) | 575 | (93.9%) |
| | susp.malig.appear. | 60( 9.8%) | 13 | ( 2.1%) |
| | malig.appear. | 12( 1.9%) | 24 | ( 3.9%) |

of histological type of carcinoma by echography was also
effective, particularly in the case of scirrhous ( 83% )
and medullary tubular carcinoma ( 78% ). On the other
hand, on 612 cases of benign tumors, echography showed
lower false positive rate ( 6.0% ) including suspected
malignant appearance than X-ray mammography which showed
11%. Through these studies, it was confirmed that echography was useful not only for the detection of breast
cancer in the early stage but also for the differentiation
of histological type of carcinoma by careful analysis of
fine echographic images in relation to the improved image
quality.

SCREENING OF BREAST CANCER BY ECHOGRAPHY

According to the improved technological advancement
of echographic equipment and to the excellent clinical
result mentioned above, screening of breast cancer by
echography has been tried with it's various clinical
sdvantages. Various appratus for the screening use have
been developed at the Research Center and Fig.4 is the
van for breast cancer screening provided with echographic
apparatus and Fig.5 is the interior view of echographic
examination room in the screening van developed in 1975.
Screening project has been conducted in Toyama Prefecture,
Japan since 1975. Age of applicant women was principally
over 30 years old. Procedure of screening was carried out
as follows. The first step was an interview that was the

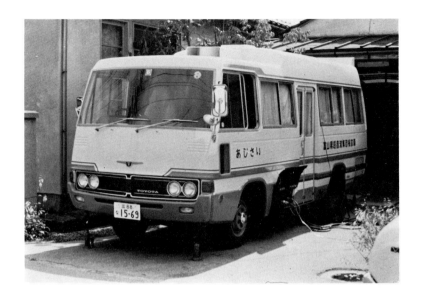

Fig.4 Van for screening of breast cancer provided with echographic equipment

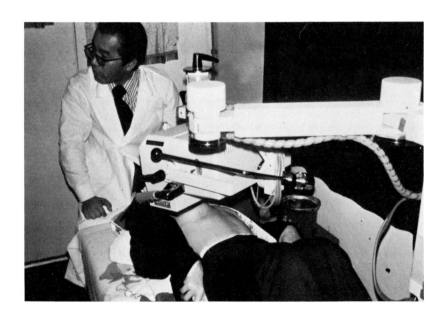

Fig.5 Interior view of echographic examination room in the screening van

check of family and individual history by public health
nurses. Then, precise inspection and palpation of the
breast was performed by doctor. Doctor marked the point
on the breast skin where any abnorml slight findings including lump and induration were palpated. Immediately after
that, echographic examinations were carried out at 15X5cm
area of the breast around the mark indicated by doctor by
nine serial parallel echograms with 5mm interval by sonographers. Automatic recording of echograms by camera was
completed within 30 second and echographic examination of
both breast was performed within 3 or 4 minute. The interpretation and judgment of echograms were performed by
double check system of two doctors and the result of echographic screening were classified into four categories.
Category I was no pathological findings, II was benign
appearance, III was suspecion of malignant appearance and
IV was malignant appearance. Women who were judged category III or IV were adviced to recieve other clinical
examinations including mammography and biopsy immediately.
During the last 6 years, total number of women who were
screened by echography were 20,323. Of these, 192 cases of
category II and 25 cases of category III and IV were
detected. Among these 25 cases, 14 cases of breast cancer
including three cases of early cancer were confirmed by
biopsy.
    The equipment and screening procedure mentioned above
are a kind of shoot examination under the guide of palpation. On the other hand, detection of allover ultrasonic
informations of the breast has been expected, particularly
for the detection of non symptomatic or non palpable cancer.
For such purpose, complete automatic properties of equipment including high speed of scanning and recording of
images will be required. Fig.6 is one of the example which
is satisfied these requests ( Syatem 1, Ausonics Co. ).
The breast is immersed freely in the water tank at prone
position and is imaged by water-pass mechanical compound
scanning modality with four focused transducers ( 4MHz )
from the bottom of the water tank. Scanning speed is slightly changed by selected number of transducer and angle of
sector scanning, but is 0.5 sec on the average. Scanning
area is 15X15cm and serial parallel echography with any
desired interval from 1mm at any direction can be recorded.
These serial echograms are recorded directly by VTR. I
tried to apply the equipment for the screening of breast
cancer in October 1981 in Tokyo after examining clinical
efficacy of this equipment at University Hospital. For the
screening use of this equipment, I selected two inside
transducers with 50 degree of sector scanning angle and
5mm interval for serial transverse echography from the
practical point of view. According to such conditions, 30
serial echograms were recorded on one side breast by VTR
within 50 sec and echographic examination of both breast
was completed within 3 or 4 minute. 641 women who were
detected abnormal findings at the first step of screening

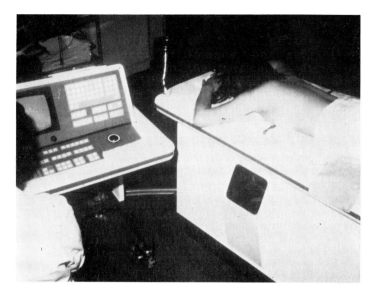

Fig.6  System 1, Ausonics Co.

by doctor's palpation were examined by this system. Of
these, 11 cases were detected as category III and IV and
were followed by other clinical examination and biopsy.
Until now, one case of breast cancer was detected from
these cases. Through the screening trial by applying
System 1, automation properties of examination and recording and other procedure were ideal, however, the problem
was the interpretation of echographic images. Data processing techniques for the interpretation of such a lot of
informations will be expected in future.

     The progress of the echographic technique for the
dete ction of breast cancer was discussed in light of
recent results obtained at my Research Center. The design
and performance of echographic apparatus introduced for
screening of breast cancer and an actual screening and it's
results were also discussed. Furthermore, application of
the equipment with automatic performance for the screening
of breast cancer was discussed and these results were very
promising together with the various advantages of diagnostic
ultrasound in future.

REFERENCES

1. Wagai,T., Tsutsumi,M. and Takeuchi,H. ( 1975 ) :
   Diagnostic ultrasound in breast diseases, Diagnostic
   Ultrasound, p. 148. Editors: Ian Donald & S. Levi,
   Kooyker Scientific Publications, Rotterdam-Netherlands

2. Wagai,T. and Tsutsumi,M. ( 1977 ) :
   Ultrasound examination of the breast, Breast Carcinoma,
   p. 325. Editor : W.W.Logan, John Wiley & Sons, New
   York
3. Wagai, T. and Tsutsumi,M. ( 1979 ) : Analytical invest-
   gation of ultrasonic breast carcinoma images in relation to the performance of equipment and histological
   structure, Report of 2nd WFUMB meeting in Miyazaki,
   p. 126
4. Tsutsumi, M. and Wagai, T. ( 1979 ) : Screening of
   breast cancer by ultrasound, p. 105, Report of 2nd
   WFUMB meeting in Miyazaki
5. Wagai, T. and Tsutsumi, M. ( 1981 ) : Echographic
   differentiation of histological structure in breast
   carcinoma, Recent advances in ultrasound diagnosis 3,
   Proceedings of the 4th European Congress on Ultrasonics
   in Medicine, p. 369, Editors : A. Kurjak and A. Kratochwil, Excerpta Medica, Amsterdam, Holland

# COMPUTERIZED, WATER IMMERSION ULTRASONOGRAPHY IN THE DIAGNOSIS OF BREAST TUMORS 1 CENTIMETER OR SMALLER IN ALL BREAST TYPES

Raul H. Matallana

*Department of Radiology, Division of Oncologic Diagnostic Radiology, University of Wisconsin Clinical Science Center, Madison, WI, U.S.A.*

The first attempt to apply ultrasound to the diagnosis of breast pathology was reported by John Wild in 1952. Wild used A mode ultrasound to distinguish between benign and malignant lesions based upon ultrasonic pattern.

However, diagnostic ultrasonography for breast disease did not become popular until improved results were obtained with the Grey Scale ultrasonic system and, more recently, with the automated ultrasound equipment specifically designed for breast diagnosis. These more advanced technologies have significantly increased the potential for accurate breast ultrasound diagnosis.

At the University of Wisconsin we have been using sequentially B mode and a real-time, small parts Doppler system since 1974. Recently, we incorporated a computerized, water-immersion automatic ultrasound system for breast scanning, introduced by the Ausonics Company, New Berlin, Wisconsin.

## MATERIALS AND METHODS

Forty patients with breast carcinomas of 1 centimeter or less, with and without calcifications, were retrospectively evaluated sequentially with physical examination (palpation), mammography and ultrasound. The breast mammography density of these cases corresponds to types P-2 and DY according to Wolfe's classification.

Thirty-five of the 40 patients were examined by Doppler B mode ultrasound, and the remaining five by water-immersion ultrasound.

Considerations for Ultrasonic diagnosis:

As previously stated by several authors, among them Teixedor and Kazam, Scott I. Fields, Jellins, Kossof and Kobayashi, the major criteria used for breast ultrasonic diagnosis are:

1. Outline of a mass.
2. Border (thick and irregular margins are associated with tumor invasion, thin borders represent abrupt interface between the tumor itself and the normal breast tissue).
3. Presence, absence and/or homogeneity of internal echos.
4. Characteristics of the posterior wall.
5. Extent of through transmission (shadowing, enhancement, or no alteration).

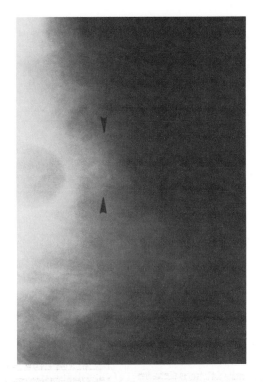

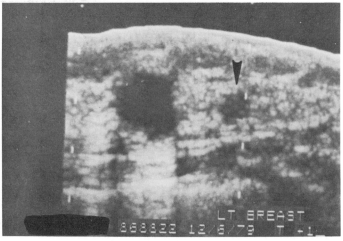

Fig.1 Xerography: Cluster of subareolar malignant calcifications without mammographic mass lesions.

6. Disruption of normal architecture.
7. Nature of the surrounding tissues.

We agree with those authors, who state that a combination of factors rather than any single factor leads to a sonographic diagnosis.

However, we believe that the most reliable criteria are:

Solid Mass

Disruption of normal architecture.
Irregular and thick echogenic borders.
Attenuation.

RESULTS

All 40 cases were sequentially evaluated in the following order: clinical history, physical examination, mammography, and ultrasound. The information from each of these methods was then evaluated and compared.

ACCURACY OF NONINVASIVE TECHNIQUES IN DIAGNOSING BREAST TUMORS
1 CM OR SMALLER

| METHOD | # PATIENTS DIAGNOSED/TOTAL # PATIENTS (% ACCURACY) |
|---|---|
| Palpation | 12/40  (30%) |
| Mammography | 34/40  (85%) |
| Ultrasound: | |
|    Doppler B Mode | 22/35  (62.8%) |
|    Water Immersion | 4/5  (80%) |
| All Methods Combined | 36/40  (90%) |

Physical examination detected 12 cases, for a 30% diagnostic accuracy. Mammography correctly diagnosed 34 cases for an 85% accuracy. Ultrasound (combining data from both ultrasound methods used), 26 cases were detected for a 65% accuracy. Using the Doppler type and B mode ultrasound systems, 22 tumors out of 35 were detected (62.8%), and four out of five patients evaluated with the new water-immersion automatic ultrasound system were accurately diagnosed (80%). The combined results of physical examination, mammography and ultrasound yielded a correct diagnosis in 36 out of 40 patients (90%).

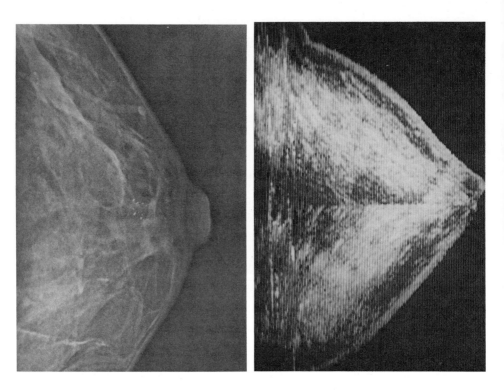

Fig.2 By-attenuation, the cluster of calcifications produce distinct subareolar shadow on automatic high resolution breast ultrasound (Ausonics, Part 1 Model).

Two cases showed questionable findings by mammography and ultrasound, but were positively identified with physical examination. In two other cases, mammography and ultrasound were negative and physical examination revealed questionable findings.

## DISCUSSION

Although the number of patients evaluated for this report is small, the results strongly suggest that ultrasonography, especially the newer water immersion system, can offer valuable information in the diagnosis of small (less than 1 centimeter) lesions of the breast, especially when used in conjunction with mammography and palpation. It is well established that mammography often cannot distinguish small lesions in dense breast tissue. However, high resolution ultrasound not only can distinguish small lesions with or without calcifications, in dense breast tissue, it also does not expose the patient to ionizing radiation.

Sonographically, an infiltrating stellate tumor mass has irregular borders and a weaker or absent posterior wall. Direct contact sonography can effectively diagnose the knobby type of tumor with multiple nodularity which has nonhomogeneous internal echos, if present. There might be minor or no attenuation of the posterior wall, depending upon the presence or not of a significant desmoplastic reaction.

However, the sonographic diagnosis may be less clear with a well-circumscribed carcinoma. With such tumors, the radiologists should note that through transmission is consistently diminished, a sonographic characteristic which makes ultrasonic evaluation of mammographically questionable masses clearly valuable in the differential diagnosis.

Ultrasonography, especially the newer water-immersion type is a simple, noninvasive procedure that provides valuable additional information to palpation and mammography that can also diminish the need for biopsies by distinguishing between malignant and non-malignant lesions. Although mammography remains the single, most sensitive diagnostic method for detecting early breast cancer, ultrasonography offers a nonionizing, complementary approach for detecting small lesions in dense breast tissue, thereby significantly enhancing diagnostic accuracy in women of all ages.

## REFERENCES

1.    Jellius and Kossoff:  Ultrasound in Medicine and Biology. Vol. I, pp. 393-404, 1975.

2.    Wolfe, John N:  Radiology, 131: 267-268, April 1979.

3.    Kobayashi, T:  Journal of Clinical Ultrasound. 7:471-479, December 1979.

# THE ROLE OF STANDARDIZED ECHOGRAPHY IN THE DIAGNOSIS AND MANAGEMENT OF CANCER OF THE EYE, ORBIT AND PERIORBITAL REGION

Karl C. Ossoinig

*Department of Ophthalmology, The University of Iowa, Iowa City, IA 52242, U.S.A.*

## WHAT IS STANDARDIZED ECHOGRAPHY?

Standardized Echography is by far the most effective and accurate ultrasonic method used to diagnose and differentiate tumors of the eye, orbit and periorbital region. It is based on an A-scan method that is specifically designed for tissue diagnosis, and is standardized in both instrumentation and examination techniques. This standardized A-scan is complemented by contact real-time B-scan and Doppler techniques.

The standardized A-scan (Kretztechnik 7200 MA principle) utilizes a small, cylindrical 8 MHz probe with a crystal diameter of 5 mm. A narrow-band receiver is optimally tuned to 8 MHz, and provides a maximal signal-to-noise ratio, thus permitting the very high system sensitivities necessary for the display of weakly scattering tissues. The narrow-band receiver also enhances the weakening of echo signals caused by absorption in the tissues so that the more complicated and less efficient use of higher frequencies to differentiate tissues with varying sound absorption values is not necessary. The various absorption values become easily recognizable from the different angles 'kappa' of the tissue echograms (see Fig. 1). The signal processing utilizes S-shaped amplification characteristics with a specific distribution of dynamic range (33 db between 5% and 95% high spikes; 16 db between 2% and 57% high signals). This S-shaped amplification represents the best possible compromise between the opposite and extreme properties of linear and logarithmic amplifiers (none of which are suited for tissue differentiation). The S-shaped amplification permits optimal enhancement of acoustic differences between tissues and, at the same time, allows simultaneous evaluation of thick tissue layers (up to 100 mm thickness in tissues that absorb little acoustic energy, and up to 20 mm thickness in tissues which absorb strongly). In addition to the specific amplifier characteristics, the signal processing provides a special ratio between display height and horizontal screen expansion, specifically strong high-frequency filtering, specific limiting of amplitudes and many other features, all of which, through years of intensive experimental and clinical work, have been found

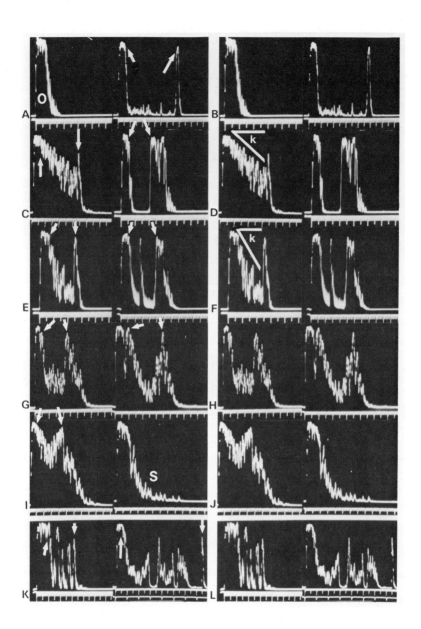

to optimally enhance the acoustic differences between different tissues.

For standardized echography, the Kretztechnik 7200 MA standardized A-scan and a real-time contact B-scan unit (we use the Ocuscan 400 of Sonometrics) are used together: both instruments are placed on a mobile cart so that standardized echography can be performed in the office, at the patient's bedside and in the operating room. By simply alternating between the A-scan and B-scan probes, and observing the A-scan and B-scan screens, a quick and effective combination of A- and B-scan techniques can be utilized. This arrangement is necessary because no single instrument with optimal A-scan and B-scan displays is presently available. A-scan and B-scan require different probes and signal processing for effective use. Instruments that provide simultaneous A- and B-scan displays have so far emphasized the B-scan component and neglected the A-scan which is of crucial importance for tissue diagnosis.

Both A- and B-scan methods are applied in a dynamic fashion. The ultrasonic beam or acoustic section is shifted and angled continuously through the tissues while the examiner observes the resulting changes in the display on the screen.

Ophthalmic ultrasound differs remarkably from echographic methods used in other areas of the body: the use of higher frequencies, i.e., 8 MHz or more, is possible because of the small extension of the ocular structures and the fact that the eye ball serves as an acoustic window allowing easy access to the deeper orbital tissues. On the other hand, this use of higher frequencies provides a different basis (higher level of resolution) for tissue differentiation than that utilized, for example, in abdominal examinations. The clearly defined boundaries of the orbits

---

←

Fig. 1. Paraocular A-scan echograms which are representative for various orbital tissues. A. Normal orbital tissues; B. Orbital mucocele; C. Cavernous hemangioma of the adult type; D. Serous cyst; E. Carcinoid metastatic to lacrimal gland; F. A-V fistula (dilated superior orbital vein with arterialized blood flow indicated by the blurred blood spikes); G. Encapsulated pseudotumor; H. Poorly outlined pseudotumor (low V-shape); I. Metastatic carcinoma (high V-shape); J. Sclerosing pseudotumor; K. Lymphangioma; L. Periorbital malignancy (carcinoma of the maxillary sinus). The arrows point at the surface signals that outline most of the tissue echograms (except for the normal orbital tissues (O) and the sclerosing pseudotumor (S), which are both acoustically diffuse). The high spike within the echogram of the dilated superior orbital vein (A-V fistula) is the vessel wall (sound beam aimed across a meandering portion of that dilated vessel). Note the difference between these different tissue echograms in regard to average spike height, in distribution of spike height determining the angle kappa (k) or V-shape of the echogram, and in border signals.

(outlined by bone) and of the globe (outlined by sclera)
allow the easy use of A-scan for displaying various acoustic properties of ocular tissues. Thus, tissue diagnosis
in ophthalmology, in spite of the great variety of tumors
occurring in this area (more than 150 different tissue or
lesion types), has become quite successful with the aid of
ultrasound.

However, it should be pointed out that methods other
than 'standardized echography' are employed in ophthalmology, and that 'ophthalmic ultrasound' is not a homogeneous
method per se. Standardized echography provides by far the
most reliable, accurate and detailed results in ophthalmic
tissue diagnosis, and will, therefore, be the only method
discussed in this article.

ECHOGRAPHIC TISSUE DIFFERENTIATION

Standardized A-scan is used to detect or rule out lesions
in the eye, orbit and periorbital region. Once a lesion is
detected, special A-scan, B-scan and Doppler techniques are
employed to localize, measure and differentiate the lesion.

Orbital and Periorbital Tumors:

Quantitative A-scan echography evaluates the internal structure, reflectivity and sound attenuation within a lesion.
Topographic B-scans and A-scans are used to determine the
borders, shape and location of a lesion. Kinetic A-scans
and B-scans are then employed to determine the vascularity,
mobility and consistency of the lesion. Table 1 lists the
various possibilities of these nine acoustic key criteria
that allow the differentiation of more than 60 lesions or
groups of conditions within the orbit and periorbital region. By employing the standardized quantitative, topographic and kinetic echographic techniques, and using check
lists like the one for orbital differentiation shown in
Table 1, even a technician can differentiate ocular lesions
on the basis of well established combinations of acoustic
criteria that characterize a lesion or a group of conditions.
Work is under way to create a computer program based on
these criteria to facilitate clinical differential diagnoses, and to gather data to allow the prediction of the pro-
babilities of those diagnoses.

Figure 1 displays a number of standardized A-scan echograms representative for various orbital tissues. Note the
differences in spike height, which range from zero (serous
cyst) to extremely high (normal orbital tissues). There are
differences in internal structure which is, for instance,
irregular in lymphangiomas and periorbital malignancies
(mostly carcinomas of the sinuses), but regular in most
other lesions. The angle kappa, which is the angle between
the baseline and a line through the centers or peaks of
tissue signals (excluding the surface spikes), indicates
whether a tissue is absorbing ultrasonic energy strongly

Table 1. Echographic Data Checklist for Differential Diagnosis of Orbital Mass Lesions.
The nine acoustic key criteria, i.e., structure, reflectivity, sound absorption, borders, shape, location, vascularity, mobility and consistency, as well as other acoustic criteria, e.g. bony defects, are to be evaluated with quantitative, topographic and kinetic echography. In this case, the acoustic properties typical of a cavernous hemangioma of the adult type have been checked off.

PROGRAM 1: ORBITAL and PERIORBITAL MASS LESIONS[*]

PATIENT'S NAME: . . . . . . . . . . . . . . . . . . . . . . . .
           (last name)         (first name) (middle initial)

BIRTH DATE: . . . . . . . . . . . . DATE OF EXAMINATION: . . . . . . .

HOSPITAL NO.: . . . . . . . . . . ECHOGRAPHY NO.: 0- . . . . . . . .

## I. QUANTITATIVE ECHOGRAPHY

### INTERNAL STRUCTURE

Regular:
1. ☑ homogeneous
     ☐ heterogeneous (e.g. honeycomb-like)
2. ☐ septa with fluid-filled spaces
3. ☐ septa in solid tissue
4. ☐ unknown
5. ☐ Irregular
6. ☐ Borderline

### REFLECTIVITY

Regular (homogeneous):
7. ☐ no reflectivity (0%)
8. ☐ extremely low (0%-5%)
9. ☐ low (5%-40%)
10. ☐ medium (40%-60%)
11. ☑ high (60%-95%)
12. ☐ extremely high (95%-100%)

Regular (heterogeneous):
13. ☐ extremely low to low (1%-40%) with high-reflective septa
14. ☐ low (5%-40%) with low-to-medium-reflective septa
15. ☐ medium (40%-60%) with high-reflective septa
16. ☐ Irregular
17. ☐ Borderline

### SOUND ATTENUATION

Direct evaluation:
18. ☐ no or negative angle kappa
19. ☐ small angle kappa (<30°)
20. ☑ 45° angle kappa
21. ☐ medium angle kappa (30°-60°)
22. ☐ large angle kappa (>60°)

Indirect evaluation:
23. ☐ not evaluated
24. ☐ dense shadow
25. ☐ mild shadow
26. ☐ no shadow
27. ☐ very strong internal multiple signals
28. ☐ strong internal multiple signals
29. ☐ weak internal multiple signals
30. ☐ no internal multiple signals
31. ☐ unknown

## II. TOPOGRAPHIC ECHOGRAPHY

### LESION BORDERS

Regular:
32. ☐ unknown definition and course
33. ☐ diffuse (bordered by normal structures only)

[*]Check all relevant boxes, or all possible alternatives if undecided, in each group of acoustic criteria.

Table 1, continued.

34. ☐ poorly outlined (infiltrative)
35. ☑ well outlined (encapsulated)
36. ☐ sharply outlined (cyst
wall)
37. ☐ smooth
38. ☑ bumpy
39. ☐ lobulated
40. ☐ Irregular
41. ☐ Undetermined

SHAPE

Regular:
42. ☐ round
43. ☑ round to oval
44. ☐ oval
45. ☐ spindle-shaped
46. ☐ disc-shaped
47. ☐ thin
48. ☐ shell-like
49. ☐ multilobulated
50. ☐ poorly defined
51. ☐ Irregular
52. ☐ Undetermined

NUMBER OF LESIONS:

53. ☑ unilateral - one lesion
54. ☐ unilateral - multiple
lesions
55. ☐ bilateral - one lesion
each orbit
56. ☐ bilateral - multiple
lesions (>2)

LOCATION

57. ☐ within optic-nerve
sheaths*
58. ☐ within muscle sheaths**

Within muscle cone:
59. ☑ within muscle cone only
60. ☑ with superotemporal extension
61. ☑ with inferotemporal extension
62. ☐ with superonasal extension
63. ☐ with inferonasal extension

*Turn to Program 2
**Turn to Program 3

With Tenon's Space:
64. ☐ only at muscle insertion(s)
65. ☐ extensive (between muscles)
66. ☐ extensive (including optic-
nerve area)
67. ☐ only in optic nerve area
68. ☐ location within Tenon's
space not specified

Peripheral orbit:
69. ☐ anterior orbit
70. ☐ medium orbit
71. ☐ posterior orbit
72. ☐ superotemporal
73. ☐ inferotemporal
74. ☐ superonasal
75. ☐ inferonasal
76. ☐ Orbital apex
77. ☐ Lacrimal gland area
78. ☐ Lacrimal drainage system
(sac region)
79. ☐ Most of orbit

Sinuses:
80. ☐ frontal sinus
81. ☐ ethmoidal sinus
82. ☐ maxillary sinus
83. ☐ sphenoidal sinus
84. ☐ Nose

Retroorbitally:
85. ☐ optic canal
86. ☐ superior fissure
87. ☐ brain
88. ☐ skull
89. ☐ Roof
90. ☐ Floor
91. ☐ Medial wall
92. ☐ Temporal bone and fossa

Anterior to orbit:
93. ☐ epibulbar
94. ☐ conjunctival
95. ☐ upper lid
96. ☐ lower lid
97. ☐ brow region
98. ☐ cheek
99. ☐ dorsum nasi
100. ☐ elsewhere

Orbital involvement:
101. ☐ none
102. ☑ orbit only
103. ☐ primarily orbit

Table 1, continued.

104. ☐ secondarily orbit
105. ☐ unspecified

Bony Defects:
106. ☑ none
107. ☐ partial
108. ☐ total
109. ☐ regular and roundish
110. ☐ - single small
111. ☐ - single large
112. ☐ - multiple
113. ☐ irregular
114. ☐ - single
115. ☐ - multiple
116. ☐ bone thinning
117. ☐ bone excavation
118. ☐ bone protrusion
119. ☐ - localized
120. ☐ - diffuse
121. ☐ questionable defect

SIZE (maximum diameter):
122. ☐ <2 mm
123. ☐ 2-5 mm
124. ☐ 6-10 mm
125. ☑ 11-15 mm
126. ☑ 16-30 mm
127. ☑ 31-50 mm
128. ☐ >50 mm

III. KINETIC ECHOGRAPHY

VASCULARITY

129. ☑ no blood flow

Amount of blood flow:
130. ☐ unknown
131. ☐ all blood flow

Partial blood flow:
132. ☐ sporadic
133. ☐ moderate
134. ☐ extensive
135. ☐ questionable (±)

Quality of blood flow:
136. ☐ unknown
137. ☐ arterial
138. ☐ venous
139. ☐ mixed

Type of blood flow:
140. ☐ unknown
141. ☐ directional (narrow)
142. ☐ directional (broad)
143. ☐ diffuse
144. ☐ directional (broad) or
     diffuse
145. ☐ questionable

MOBILITY

146. ☐ immobile
147. ☐ questionable
148. ☐ unknown
149. ☑ mobile toward globe
150. ☑ mobile toward bone
151. ☑ mobile toward muscles
152. ☑ mobile toward optic nerve
153. ☑ mobile toward other struc-
     tures
154. ☐ mobile with globe
155. ☐ mobile with muscles
156. ☐ mobile with optic nerve
157. ☐ mobile with other structures

CONSISTENCY

158. ☐ Unknown
159. ☐ Poorly defined

Non-Compressible:
160. ☐ rock-hard
161. ☐ hard
162. ☐ not specified

Compressible:
163. ☐ minimally compressible
     (firm)
164. ☐ slightly compressible
165. ☐ soft
166. ☑ delayed compressibility
167. ☐ not specified

Collapsible:
168. ☐ promptly collapsible
169. ☐ delayed collapsibility
170. ☐ not specified

or weakly. Hemangioma of the adult type, for instance, produces a medium angle kappa, whereas this angle is very small (minimal sound absorption) in pseudotumors. Differences in borders indicated by the appearance of the maximum surface spikes on the right of the tissue echograms can be noted in the echograms: sharply rising (with very few high-frequency knots visible on the left ascending limb of the surface spike), double-peaked spikes are typical for cyst walls (see serous cyst in Fig. 1); steeply rising, high, narrow, mostly single-peaked spikes are characteristic of well encapsulated lesions (e.g., in cavernous hemangioma); poorly outlined (infiltratively growing) tumors show broad, multi-peaked surface spikes and a V-shaped echogram (e.g., carcinoma); and diffuse lesions lack a clear surface signal altogether (e.g., sclerosing pseudotumor).

There are several other acoustic criteria which cannot be documented in a single echogram photo. They are evaluated during the dynamic examination of the patient by directly observing the screen display. These kinetic data add greatly to the differential diagnostic process.

Table 2. Echographic key criteria of hemangiomas of the adult and infant types (also see Table 1). Note that these two different tumors do not have a single acoustic property in common.

| | HEMANGIOMAS | |
| | Cavernous (adult type) | Mixed Cavernous/Capillary (infant type) |
| --- | --- | --- |
| INTERNAL STRUCTURE | Regular heterogeneous: (septa separating fluid-filled spaces) | Irregular |
| REFLECTIVITY | High (spike height is 80-90% of display height at tissue sensitivity) | Irregular (high and low) |
| SOUND ABSORPTION | medium angle kappa ($\tilde{-}45^{o}$) | Minimal |
| BORDERS | Well-outlined (encapsulated) with bumpy surface | Well-outlined (encapsulated) but irregular |
| SHAPE | Round or oval | Irregular |
| LOCATION | Typically within muscle cone | Typically in superior anterior orbit |
| VASCULARITY | No blood flow (stagnant blood) | Massive, pulsatile blood flow |
| MOBILITY | Mobile toward all structures | Immobile toward surrounding structures |
| CONSISTENCY | Hard (with delayed compressibility) | Soft |

Rarely, a lesion can be diagnosed from a single specific criterion, as is the case, for instance, in arteriovenous fistulas of the cavernous sinus that drain through an orbit. The spontaneous and continuous, fast, vertical, flickering motion of all lesion spikes indicates fast (arterialized) blood flow within the dilated superior ophthalmic vein (see Fig. 1), and allows the examiner to make a definite diagnosis of A-V fistula, often within the first twenty seconds of an examination.

Usually, the combination of several or all of the nine main acoustic criteria is necessary to separate a particular lesion from all others. Cavernous hemangiomas of the adult type, for example, differ in each single main criterion from hemangiomas of the infant type (Table 2), but have at least one criterion, i.e., the high reflectivity, in common with metastatic carcinomas (Table 3). These most frequent types of orbital carcinomas can be identified reliably and clearly with standardized echography on the basis of several acoustic features. Adenoid cystic carcinoma of the lacrimal gland, an example of the rare primary orbital cancer, also provides typical echographic patterns (Table 4), which allow its separation from most other lesions. However, this lacrimal-gland tumor differs from the benign epithelial tumor of this organ, the so-called benign mixed tumor of the lacrimal gland in only one major acoustic criterion (i.e., reflectivity), and that to a small degree only (Table 4). Nevertheless, standardized echography is still very helpful in suspecting, if not indicating, the presence, and consequently influencing the management of, this highly malignant tumor.

Sometimes, it is not possible with today's technology and knowledge to differentiate individual lesions within a larger group of conditions. The largest such group is

Table 3. Echographic key criteria of carcinomas, metastatic to the orbit (excluding the form of metastatic carcinoma that grows expansively within muscle sheaths)

| | Carcinoma, Metastatic to the Orbit |
|---|---|
| INTERNAL STRUCTURE | Regular |
| REFLECTIVITY | High (60-90% spike height), lowest in center (V-shaped echogram) |
| SOUND ABSORPTION | Minimal |
| BORDERS | Poorly outlined (infiltrative growth) enhancing the V-shape of the echogram |
| SHAPE | Roundish or poorly defined |
| LOCATION | Typically in superior orbit |
| VASCULARITY | No blood flow |
| MOBILITY | Immobile ('dead' looking pattern) |
| CONSISTENCY | Hard |

Table 4. Echographic key criteria of adenoid-cystic carcinoma and of benign mixed tumor of lacrimal gland

| | LACRIMAL GLAND TUMORS | |
| | Adenoid-cystic carcinoma | Benign mixed tumor |
| --- | --- | --- |
| INTERNAL STRUCTURE | Regular, slightly heterogeneous (medium high septa in solid tissue) | Regular, slightly heterogeneous (medium high septa in solid tissue) |
| REFLECTIVITY | Medium high (50-60% spike height) | High to extremely high (80-100% spike height) |
| SOUND ABSORPTION | Medium (medium angle kappa | Medium or strong (medium to large angle kappa) |
| BORDERS | Well outlined (encapsulated) | Well outlined (encapsulated) |
| SHAPE | Round to oval | Round to oval |
| LOCATION | Lacrimal gland area | Lacrimal gland area |
| VASCULARITY | No blood flow | No blood flow |
| MOBILITY | Immobile | Immobile |
| CONSISTENCY | Hard or firm | Hard or firm |

Note the echographic similarity of these two tumors (except for reflectivity). The carcinoma may produce partial or total bony defects in later stages of the disease

'encapsulated cellular tumors', which most frequently encompasses lymphomas and inflammatory pseudotumors (and, therefore, is usually referred to as the 'lymphoma/pseudotumor group'), but may also include sarcoidosis or even, with some mild vascularization, extremely rare hemangiomatous tumors such as hemangioendotheliomas and hemangiopericytomas. Thus, echographic differential diagnosis does not replace diagnostic biopsies in a number of cases. But even in these cases, standardized echography is essential for the planning of an optimal surgical approach by informing the surgeon, for instance, whether an excisional or partial biopsy is indicated; these procedures often require totally different surgical approaches ranging from a small skin incision in the upper or lower lids to major bone resections during lateral or frontal orbitotomies. In cases where partial biopsy is indicated, the echographic findings aid in the selection of the best location for the procedure (Fig. 2).

Another application of standardized echography is the preparation of orbital cancer for radiotherapy. With other diagnostic procedures, such as computerized tomography, it is often difficult to accurately localize orbital lesions

Table 5. Echographic key criteria* and other acoustic properties of malignant melanoma of the choroid and ciliary body, and of some more frequently encountered pseudomelanomas

| | Malignant Melanoma of the Choroid | Choroidal Nevus | Metastatic Carcinoma | Atypical Disciform Lesion | Choroidal Hemangioma |
|---|---|---|---|---|---|
| *INTERNAL STRUCTURE | Regular | Irregular | Irregular | Irregular | Regular |
| *REFLECTIVITY | Low-to-medium (2-60% spike height) | Medium-to-high | Medium-to-high | Medium-to-high | High-to-extremely high (85-100% spike height) |
| *CONSISTENCY | Solid | Solid | Solid | At least partially solid | Solid |
| *VASCULARITY | Blood flow (+ to +++) | None | Usually none | None or minimal | None |
| *SHAPE | Variable (specific only when mushroom-shaped) | Relatively flat (never mushroom-shaped) | Variable (extremely rarely mushroom-shaped) | Variable (never mushroom-shaped) | Flat to dome-shaped (never mushroom-shaped) |
| SCLERAL INFILTRATION | Possible | None | None | None | None |
| EXTRAOCULAR GROWTH | Possible | None | None | None | None |

Note that the malignant melanoma as well as the pseudomelanomas listed in this table have a solid consistency. This acoustic key criterion, however, becomes very important in the differential diagnosis of other (exudative) lesions such as subchoroidal hemorrhage, which also may mimic malignant melanoma clinically.

Date:           3/5/81
Name:           S.K.
Hospital No.:   81-0252418

Clinical Impression:
ORBITAL MASS
OS

Echography No.: 0-81-579

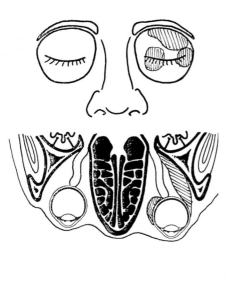

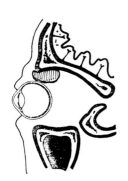

OS: multiple, regularly structured, low reflective mass lesions which absorb ultrasound only minimally. The lesions are well encapsulated and affect the lateral rectus muscle which is markedly swollen, the nasal posterior episcleral (sub-Tenon's) space, and the superior anterior orbit between the 11 and 2 o'clock meridians (including the lacrimal gland). The muscle lesion is spindle-shaped, the episcleral lesion is shell-like in shape, and the superior anterior lesion is roundish to oval with a slightly bumpy surface. None of the lesions are vascularized, and they are all hard. The episcleral lesion is mobile with the globe; the muscle lesion moves forward and backward in the orbit with eye movements; the superior anterior lesion is immobile. The maximum thickness of the lateral rectus muscle is 8.2 mm, as compared to the normal size of the right lateral rectus muscle which has a maximum thickness of 4.6 mm. The maximum thickness of the episcleral lesion is 3.5 mm; it extends between the 7 o'clock and 10:30 meridians from the equator to the posterior pole. The superior anterior lesion has a maximum sagittal extension of 18.0 mm and a maximum thickness of 7.7 mm in the 1:30 meridian. The lesion protrudes forward the most in the 1:30 meridian, where its anterior surface lies about 3 mm in front of the bony orbital rim. No bony defect detected.

Diagnosis: Lesions of the pseudotumor/lymphoma group, most likely pseudotumor because of multiple lesions in one orbit.

Best site for biopsy is 1:30 meridian below brow region.

Fig. 2. See the text on the actual Figure 2.

340

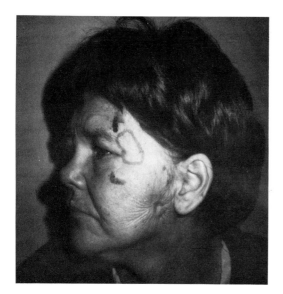

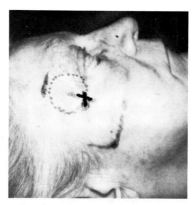

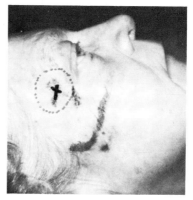

Fig. 3. Patient (illustrated at left) with metastases from scirrhous breast carcinoma to the left orbit and cheek prior to radiation therapy. The projection of the outline of the orbital tumor mass as evaluated with echography is drawn on the skin, and is the basis for the placement of the radiation field (anterior marks of the field are also seen on the skin of the patient). On the right, another patient is seen who was irradiated for carcinoid metastatic to her right lacrimal gland area. The top picture shows the original placement of the radiation field with its center (cross mark) placed at the lower edge of the tumor outlined with echography after the first radiation session. The picture below shows the corrected radiation field used for the rest of the radiotherapy (note that the center of the radiation field now coincides with the center of the tumor).

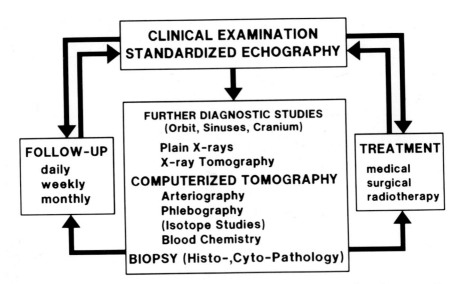

| CLINICAL EXAMINATION |
| STANDARDIZED ECHOGRAPHY |

**FOLLOW-UP**
daily
weekly
monthly

**FURTHER DIAGNOSTIC STUDIES**
(Orbit, Sinuses, Cranium)

**Plain X-rays**
**X-ray Tomography**
**COMPUTERIZED TOMOGRAPHY**
**Arteriography**
**Phlebography**
**(Isotope Studies)**
**Blood Chemistry**
**BIOPSY (Histo-,Cyto-Pathology)**

**TREATMENT**
medical
surgical
radiotherapy

Fig. 4. Standardized echography and the clinical examination are the primary tools to screen orbits for mass lesions. Standardized echography also plays a central role in identifying, localizing and measuring a tumor in this region, and thus directly or indirectly aids in the treatment and follow-up of such conditions. Standardized echography is also the most effective and economical method for indicating the selective use of further diagnostic tests, particularly and most frequently computerized tomography. (Reproduced from Neuro-Ophthalmology, 1982, Vol. 2., Editors: S. Lessell and J.T.W. van Dalen. Excerpta Medica, Amsterdam).

scheduled for radiotherapy. By marking the exact borders and their projections to the surface of the skin in a dynamic examination, standardized echography helps to optimally employ radiation therapy (Fig. 3). Through its extensive differential-diagnostic capabilities, standardized echography is also very helpful in planning other diagnostic procedures, e.g., computerized tomography, plain X-rays or blood studies. Figure 4 illustrates and explains the important clinical role of standardized echography in the diagnosis and management of orbital lesions.

Intraocular Tumors:

Malignant melanoma of the choroid and ciliary body is the primary (malignant) intraocular tumor seen in adults. With standardized echography, more than 95% of malignant melanomas can be diagnosed accurately and differentiated from other tumors and pseudotumors that clinically may mimic melanoma. Figure 5 illustrates standardized A- and B-scan echograms typical of malignant melanoma of the choroid and ciliary body. Table 5 presents the key acoustic criteria and other acoustic properties of malignant melanomas on which

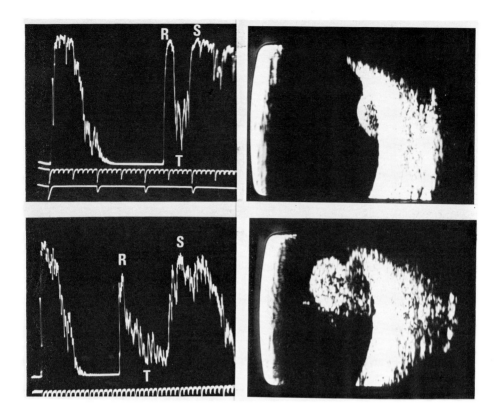

Fig. 5. A-scan and B-scan echograms of two cases of malignant melanoma of the choroid. The A-scans represent the two most frequently found, different echographic types of this tumor: the top echogram shows Type I with a very high and broad surface spike (R representing the surfaces of retina and tumor) and low internal reflectivity (T representing the tumor). The tumor spikes show about equal height (no angle kappa). S scleral surface at the base of the tumor. The bottom A-scan echogram shows a different type of melanoma: the surface spike is not as high and is narrow (R - the left peak represents the slightly elevated retina, whereas the highest peak indicates the tumor surface). The tumor spikes begin at a low-to-medium height and continuously decrease toward the right indicating a medium sized angle kappa (T). This type II malignant melanoma is the most frequently seen. The two B-scan echograms illustrate the different shapes malignant melanomas may assume. Only the mushroom shape shown in the bottom echogram is a B-scan sign specific for malignant melanoma.

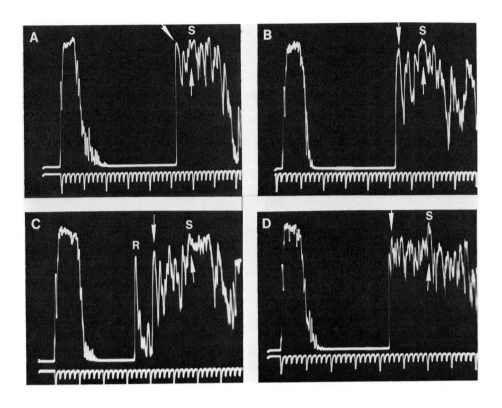

Fig. 6. A-scan echograms of more frequently encountered pseudomelanomas that may clinically mimic melanoma. Arrows point at the surface
signals and outline the pseudomelanomas; R - detached retina; S -
sclera; A choroidal nevus; B - disciform macula degeneration; C -
carcinoma metastatic to the choroid; D - choroidal hemangioma.
Note that these lesion echograms differ from the melanoma patterns by
their spike height or by the irregularity of their internal structure,
or by both of these criteria.

Fig. 7. A-scan echograms on the left represent cases that appeared
to be suspicious for malignant melanoma during the first examination
(center) or consistent with pseudomelanoma (nevus or metastatic carcinoma at top; disciform lesion at bottom). Follow-up examinations
clarified these three cases (echograms on the right). The top and
center echograms on the right are clear-cut melanoma patterns; this
diagnosis was later confirmed histologically. Note that neither tumor had grown much, but had changed internally to low reflectivity

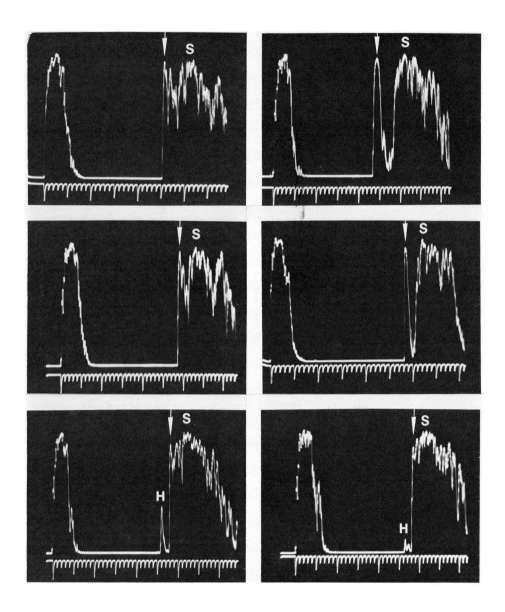

and now showed marked vascularity as documented during a dynamic examination. The bottom echogram on the right clearly shows less elevation of the lesion than on the initial examination (left bottom echogram), which confirmed the diagnosis of disciform lesion. The intervals between the first and follow-up examinations, represented by the
echograms on the left and right, were 5 months (top echograms), 4
months (center echograms) and 6 weeks (bottom echograms) respectively.
Arrows point at the surface spikes of the lesions; S - scleral signal;
H - vitreous hemorrhage.

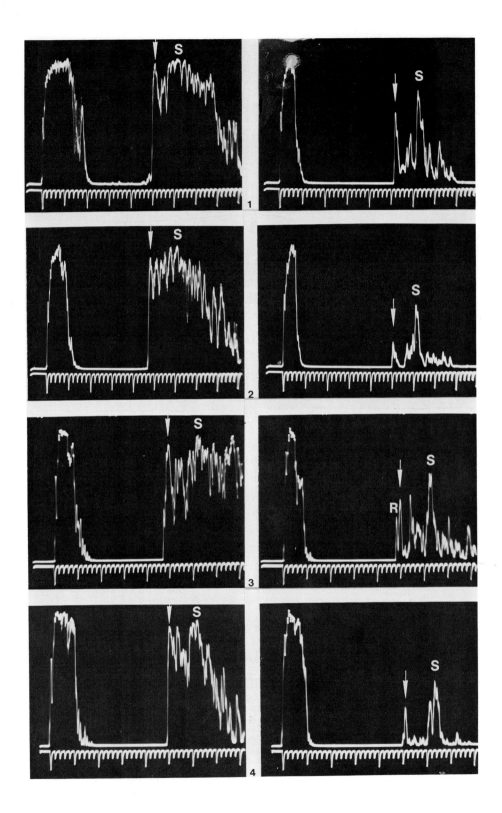

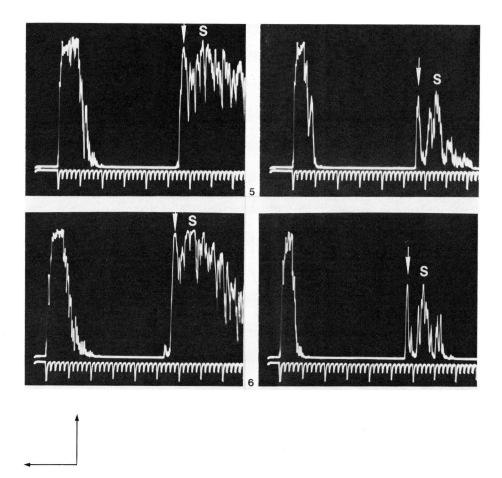

Fig. 8. Series of A-scan echograms obtained at high tissue sensitivity (left) and at low measuring sensitivity (right) in a case of atypical disciform macula degeneration. The pairs of echograms were obtained on the first examination of the patient (top), and after 6 weeks (second row), 4 months (third row), 4 weeks (fourth row), 3 months (fifth row), and 8 months (bottom) following each previous examination, respectively. The arrows indicate the surface of the mass lesion and its maximum elevation from the sclera ($\underline{S}$); $\underline{R}$ - detached retina. Unlike the case of disciform macula degeneration illustrated in Figure 7, the lesion illustrated in this figure first increased in size (without a change in its reflectivity and irregular structure, however) and then slowly regressed to a smaller elevation than that found in the initial examination over a period of almost 18 months. In a case of suspected or diagnosed 'pseudotumor', the lesion must be followed until it regresses to the less elevated scar, regardless of how long the process takes, to confirm the diagnosis and rule out an atypical malignant melanoma.

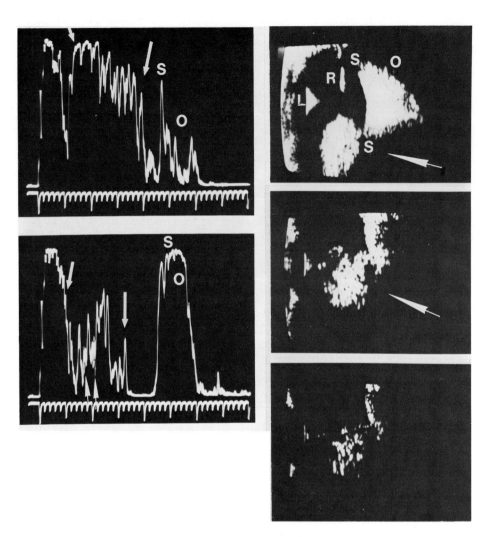

Fig. 9. A-scan and B-scan echograms of an eye with retinoblastoma. Arrows (pointing down) outline the tumor in the A-scan echograms. The tumor portion illustrated in the top echogram shows typical calcification: extremely high, slightly separate spikes at tissue sensitivity; markedly reduced height of scleral signal (S) and orbital spikes (O) caused by shadowing. Compare these signals with the very high, normal scleral and orbital echo spikes in the bottom echogram. The bottom A-scan echogram represents a non-calcified portion of the retinoblastoma which has low-to-medium reflectivity and irregular internal structure. Here arrows (pointing down) indicate blurred tumor spikes; the blurring is caused by fast, spontaneous, continuous motion of blood flowing in tumor vessels. The B-scans on the right were obtained with maximum and moderately as well as minimal system sensitivities to indicate the strong reflectivity and shadowing (arrows) of this tumor portion. R - retinal detachment next to tumor; L - signal from posterior lens surface; S - sclera. Note the dust-like distribution of the strong signals, which is obvious at the minimum system sensitivity level.

the diagnosis and differentiation are based. This table also lists the corresponding acoustic criteria of four other, more frequently encountered intraocular tumors that may be clinically confused with malignant melanoma. As can be seen from the table, it is not always possible to echographically differentiate between those pseudomelanomas. But the significant fact is that they can be differentiated safely from malignant melanomas most of the time (compare Figs. 5 and 6).

Next to ophthalmoscopy and fundus fluorescein angiography, standardized echography is the most important method today for diagnosing malignant melanoma. In almost 15% of all cases, malignant melanomas are hidden by opacities in the ocular media and cannot be evaluated safely or at all with ophthalmoscopy. In these cases, standardized echography is of the utmost importance. Even in cases with clear ocular media, standardized echography plays a major role as it provides important information about the internal structure of these tumors which cannot be obtained

Table 6. Echographic key criteria of retinoblastoma and benign pseudogliomas that may mimic malignant retinoblastoma clinically

|  | Retinoblastoma | Pseudogliomas |
|---|---|---|
| INTERNAL STRUCTURE | Irregular with typically spaced 100% high spikes (echoes from dust-like calcium deposits) | Usually regular |
| REFLECTIVITY | Extremely high (100% high spikes in at least some areas of tumor) | Low-to-medium; (except for surface spikes) |
| SOUND ABSORPTION | Extremely strong (dense shadows behind calcified portions of tumor) | Minimal |
| SHAPE | Irregular | Regular |
| VASCULARITY | + to ++ in non-calcified areas of tumor | None |
| CONSISTENCY | Partially solid and partially mobile | Usually mobile |

The acoustic key criteria of retinoblastoma are its very high internal spikes and strong shadowing, both of which are caused by the characteristic dust-like distribution of calcium deposits within portions of the tumor. Pseudogliomas may contain areas of calcification or bone formation too, but only in very late stages of the condition when eye is already phthisical (a condition not found in retinoblastoma). Also, calcification in phthisical eyes is plaque-like and thus echographically quite different from the dust-like distribution seen regularly in retinoblastoma.

from any other diagnostic source, thus adding an independent second evaluation obtained from a different perspective than that provided by the clinical examination. Standardized echography is also the best means for the accurate determination of the vertical growth of a fundus tumor, and for the early detection of scleral infiltration and extraocular growth. The latter consideration is of ever increasing importance since small malignant melanomas are frequently treated with radiation or photocoagulation. In these cases, the tumor growth may be arrested inside the eye, but tumor cells may grow through the sclera into the retrobulbar space without being noted by ophthalmoscopy. Echographic follow-up examinations are also very helpful for the management of intraocular tumors as Figures 7 and 8 illustrate.

The counterpart in children to malignant melanoma is retinoblastoma. Figure 9 illustrates, and Table 6 lists, the echographic features typical for retinoblastoma.
Table 7 indicates the most frequently encountered (benign) 'pseudogliomas' which may (and often do) mimic retinoblastoma clinically, but which can be differentiated from the malignancy with standardized echography. Table 6 contrasts the echographic findings in pseudogliomas with the acoustic criteria of retinoblastoma.

Table 7. Some more frequently encountered pseudogliomas (conditions that may mimic retinoblastoma clinically)

---

Persistent Hyperplastic Primary Vitreous (PHPV)

Retrolental Fibroplasia (RLF)

Coats' Disease

Parasites

Endophthalmitis

Retinal Dysplasia

---

As with malignant melanoma, standardized echography is a reliable and accurate method (accuracy >97%) for diagnosing malignant retinoblastoma and differentiating it from benign pseudoglioma, and thus plays an important role in addition to the clinical examination.

In summary, standardized ophthalmic echography is an essential tool for screening the orbits and eyes with opaque ocular media for the presence of a tumor, and for differentiating malignancies from benign tumors regardless of whether the ocular media are clear or opaque. Echography also helps in mapping, measuring and following up ocular tumors, and thus plays an essential role in the optimal management of cancer of the eye, orbit and periorbital region (see Fig. 4).

350

REFERENCES

Byrne, S.F. (1979): Standardized echography, part I: A-scan
   examination procedures. In: Ophthalmic Ultrasonography:
   Comparative Techniques (International Ophthalmology Clinics 19, 4), pp. 267-281. Editor: R.L. Dallow. Little,
   Brown and Co., Boston.
Ossoinig, K.C. (1979): Standardized echography: Basic principles, clinical applications and results. In: Ophthalmic Ultrasonography: Comparative Techniques (Internatio-
   nal Ophthalmology Clinics 19, 4), pp. 127-210. Editor:
   R.L. Dallow. Little, Brown and Co., Boston.
Ossoinig, K.C. (1981): Echographic differentiation of vas-
   cular tumors in the orbit. In: Ultrasonography in Ophthal-
   mology: Proceedings of the 8th SIDUO Congress (Documenta
   Ophthalmologica Proceedings Series, Volume 29), pp. 283-
   291. Editors: J.M. Thijssen and A.M. Verbeek. Dr. W.
   Junk, The Hague.
Ossoinig, K.C. (1982): Diagnostic ultrasound. In: Neuro-
   Ophthalmology, Vol. 2, Chapter 27, pp. 373-388. Editors:
   S. Lessell and J.T.W. van Dalen. Excerpta Medica, Amster-
   dam.
Till, P. and Heuff, W. (1981): Differential diagnostic re-
   sults of clinical echography in orbital tumors. In: Ul-
   trasonography in Ophthalmology: Proceedings of the 8th
   SIDUO Congress (Documenta Ophthalmologica Proceedings
   Series, Volume 29, pp. 277-282. Editors: J.M. Thijssen
   and A.M. Verbeek. Dr. W. Junk, The Hague.

# INDEX OF AUTHORS

SUBJECT INDEX

Prepared by H. Kettner, M.D., Middelburg